# ZOONOSES

## Animal Diseases That Affect Man

*By Twelve Authors*

Edited by Dr. D. E. Goodman
Clemson University, retired
Turbeville, SC, USA

Christian
Veterinary
Mission



*A Publication of Christian Veterinary Mission*

***Current Book Information at:***
**www.cvm.org**

## Raising Healthy Animals Series

Every year, thousands of people around the world struggle to survive because they don't have the right knowledge, skills and resources to care for their animals. Christian Veterinary Mission (CVM) sends veterinary professionals to live and work alongside many of these people to encourage them and provide them with not only much needed veterinary expertise, but also the hope that is only found in Christ. CVM veterinarians build lasting relationships with individuals and communities, helping them be transformed through Christ's love.

CVM, in its effort to be meaningfully involved in work in the developing world, quickly found there was little appropriate educational material available. CVM set about developing basic resource materials in animal husbandry for farmers and agricultural workers. Apparently, they met a real need, as these books have been accepted throughout the developing nations of the world.

The series of books published by Christian Veterinary Mission includes the following in order of publication:

| | |
|---|---|
| Raising Healthy Pigs * | Drugs and Their Usage |
| Raising Healthy Rabbits * | Where There Is No Animal Doctor |
| Raising Healthy Fish | Raising Healthy Horses |
| Raising Healthy Cattle | Zoonoses: Animal Diseases That Affect Humans |
| Raising Healthy Poultry *+ | Raising Healthy Honey Bees |
| Raising Healthy Goats * | Slaughter and Preservation of Meat |
| Raising Healthy Sheep | Disease and Parasite Prevention in Farm Animals |

[Also available in: * Spanish + French].

CVM fieldworkers have also developed specific training materials for the countries in which they work.

All of these books have been put together by Christian men and women; in a labor of love and service, for people in need throughout the world. It demonstrates dedication to their profession, service to humanity and a witness to their faith. We hope that they are a help to you in developing an appropriate livestock program to meet your needs. We pray God's blessing on their use.

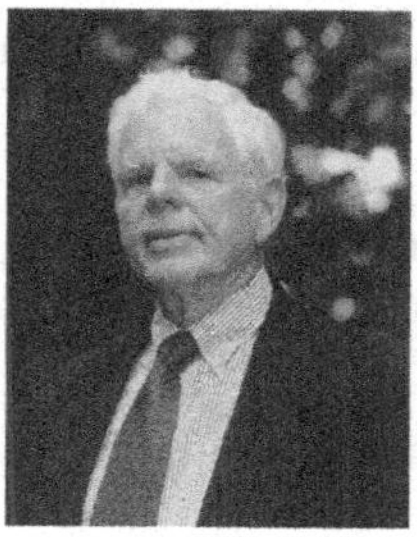

Leroy Dorminy
CVM Founder

## About the Book

Specific diseases and parasites usually affect animals within, or closely related to, the same species. Only a relatively few cross over to humans, called Zoonoses; however when this happens, the outcome can be very serious.

This book, which is a series of articles, describes a variety of zoonotic conditions and their prevention in a straightforward and practical manner.

The authors are to be commended for volunteering their time and effort to this book, and a special thanks goes to them. They have personal experience with the conditions they have written about. This is one of many books developed by Christian Veterinary Mission, with the first published in 1984. The books have been well received and are in great demand around the world. It is our sincere hope that this book will be helpful for the work in your area.

## About the Editor

Dr. D. Earle Goodman practiced for a number of years in a rural community in South Carolina, USA. He then worked as a diagnostician-epidemiologist for many years at Clemson University in South Carolina. He was also in charge of animal health programs for the state of South Carolina. Dr. Goodman was affiliated with the Air Force for thirty years, both on duty in the Middle East and North Africa, and later in the reserves. A major part of his training and responsibilities dealt with the conditions described in this book.

## *ACKNOWLEDGMENTS*

Mrs. Claire Goodman Watts for highly proficient proof-reading and editing of this book. She is an attorney in Savannah, GA, USA and former English teacher. She is the daughter of the editor.

Dr. Kelly Ward for final preparation of the book. She has a veterinary practice in rural Idaho, USA.

# Table of Contents


***About the Book*** *iii*

***About the Editor*** *iii*

**CHAPTER 1**
Rabies in Animals and Humans
*By Dr. Russell W. Currier* *1*

**CHAPTER 2**
Tuberculosis in Animals and Humans
*By Dr. Mitchell Esse* *13*

**CHAPTER 3**
Brucellosis in Animals and Humans
*By Dr. David Warner* *23*

**CHAPTER 4**
African Trypanosomes in Animals and Humans
*By Dr. David S. Peterson* *33*

**CHAPTER 5**
Venezuelan Equine Encephalomyelitis (VEE) and Related Diseases including West Nile Fever in Animals and Humans
*By Dr. Venaye P. Reese* *42*

**CHAPTER 6**
Rift Valley Fever in Animals and Humans
*By Dr. John C. Morrill* 49

**CHAPTER 7**
Anthrax in Animals and Humans
*By Dr. Keith Flanagan* 57

**CHAPTER 8**
Leptospirosis in Animals and Humans
*By Dr. John R. Cole* 67

**CHAPTER 9**
Chlamydia (Psittacosis, Ornithosis) in Birds and Humans
*By Dr. T. H. Eleazer* 75

**CHAPTER 10**
Listeriosis in Animals and Humans
*By Dr. Raymond K. Hines* 82

**CHAPTER 11**
Roundworms in Animals and Humans
*By Dr. Prema Arasu* 91

**CHAPTER 12**
Tapeworms and Trichinosis of Farm Animals which Can Cause Problems in Humans
*By Dr. Keith Flanagan* 103

***About the Authors*** **119**

CHAPTER 1

# Rabies in Animals and Humans

*By Dr. Russell W. Currier*

*Dr. Keith Sikes was the author of the original article on Rabies in Animals and Humans. He was formerly the head of the Public Health Veterinary Division in the state of Georgia. He was an outstanding authority on rabies.*

## HISTORY AND REVIEW

Rabies, also known as hydrophobia or literally "fear of water", is a viral disease affecting nervous tissue leading to an encephalitis that is invariably fatal. Its reservoir hosts are carnivorous/omnivorous animals including bats, both of which present risk of infection to humans through bites and occasionally other types of exposures. The virus is present in saliva, which is deposited in wounds, and after replication for several days and even weeks in local tissue, traverses into nerve endings and travels to the brain. After infection of the brain, it travels peripherally to various tissues including the salivary glands permitting the virus to exit and enter a new host.

Rabies was well described in classical Greek and Roman literature. These writings discussed the role of mad dogs in transmitting the disease to other dogs and humans. In the Middle Ages, large outbreaks, or epizootics, were recorded in dogs on the European continent. The use of wound cautery with red-hot irons was recognized as offering some protection.

During the 1880's, Louis Pasteur and colleagues demonstrated the predilection of the agent for the central nervous system (CNS). He was unable to cultivate any bacteria from the nervous system and stated, "one is tempted to believe that a microbe of infinite smallness, having the form neither of a bacillus nor a micrococcus is the cause." Even without being able to visualize the virus, he subsequently developed a technique to attenuate the virus through serial passage in a series of injections between dogs, monkeys, and rabbits. Later, he recognized the virus could be further attenuated by drying infected rabbit spinal cords from which he produced crude extracts that were used in vaccines. His first attempt at vaccinating a human occurred on July 6, 1885. The patient was a young boy who had been bitten 14 times by a rabid dog 60 hours earlier. He received a total of 13 inoculations of the spinal cord suspension over a ten-day period including highly virulent virus in the final doses. The child survived not only the rabid bite exposure, but the virulent virus in the final vaccine injections as well.

In the decades of the 20$^{th}$ century, inactivated nervous tissue vaccines were improved and followed by second generation vaccines developed in embryonating eggs. These vaccines were supplemented by simultaneous administration of equine-origin rabies antiserum. Third generation cell culture vaccines followed in the 1970's, complemented by introduction of human rabies immune globulins. Both products, available in the U.S. since 1980, have been protective if administered before onset of clinical disease.

### *Epidemiology*

The epizootiology of rabies is governed by strains of rabies viruses that are adapted to several host species. As a general rule, transmission of a particular strain is very efficient within a given host species, but is considerably less in other species that in turn only infrequently propagate infection to other animals or humans.

Rabies exists on all continents except Australia and Antarctica. It historically has been present in carnivorous animals, especially Canidae (primarily dogs, wolves, jackals, and foxes) but also other wildlife reservoirs including Procyonidae (e.g. raccoons), Mustelidae (e.g. skunks), Viverridae (e.g. mongooses) and Chiroptera (bats). Bat-transmitted rabies was first recognized in Spanish troops in Central America in the 16th century. Epizootics of death in livestock attributed to vampire bats were also reported. Later, the association with other bat species (e.g. insectivorous bats) was first demonstrated in Trinidad in 1931 and the U.S. in 1953.

In general, most human rabies is acquired from dogs. The World Health Organization (WHO) estimates the number of human cases of rabies globally exceeds 50,000 per year. In comparison, the U.S. has only two to three cases per year, most transmitted by bats. Recent U.S. human cases acquired from dogs have been in overseas settings where dog rabies is endemic. Accordingly, dogs present the greatest risk of rabies exposure in the landmasses of Central and South America, Africa, Asia, and the Middle East. It is comforting to note that several countries of Latin America are establishing successful control programs for urban canine rabies.

In the U.S. and Canada as well as Europe, endemic canine rabies has been eliminated, but closely related virus strains continue to exist in foxes. Other reservoirs in North America include raccoons and skunks. These three species maintain the disease with occasional "spill over" to domestic species (i.e. cats and dogs) as well as livestock (i.e. horses and cattle). The efficiency of subsequent rabies propagation cat-to-cat, dog-to-dog, and cat- or dog-to-human is low.

Bats are the other major reservoir in all land masses except Australia where even there a closely related *Lyssavirus* virus infection is found in certain frugivorous bat species and has recently been associated with a rabies-like human illness. Bats only rarely transmit rabies to terrestrial animals or people. However given the severity of the disease, any direct encounter poses some risk of exposure. Recent research concludes that bat bites may be extremely small and difficult to detect and that bat-associated strains may replicate well in dermal/cutaneous tissues where body temperature is lower. Accordingly, there is little one can do to protect against bat rabies other than avoid bats and receive immunization when a bite or other direct exposure may have occurred. In the U.S. since 1990, 32 human rabies cases have been reported with 26 acquired in the U.S. Of these, 24 were from bat sources, although available history noted suspected bat exposure in only about half the cases. Only two had a definite history of a bite.

### *Pathogenesis*

Most commonly, rabies virus is shed in saliva during the terminal stage of disease. It is in one sense a diabolical virus, since the animal is in a very agitated state (furious rabies) and will seize almost anything or other animal or human, inflict a bite(s) and deposit saliva in the tissue through the skin. The virus then goes into a prolonged localized phase including replication in various tissues such as striated muscle.

It is after the bite and during this initial replication stage that rabies virus is most vulnerable to physical removal, most optimally by immediate washing with soap and water followed by copious flushing of the wound. The presence of neutralizing antibody can also slow the virus up to several days after exposure. In the absence of these factors, the neurotropic rabies virus enters the axon of the nerve, followed by a rapid retrograde movement along nerve trunks to the CNS, and ultimately infects the brain. At this point, the blood-brain barrier prevents immune cells and rabies neutralizing antibody access to the virus. After infection of the brain, clinically distinct signs and symptoms occur with the virus then traveling centrifugally via peripheral nerves to eyes, oral and nasal cavities, and ultimately salivary glands as the usual exit point to initiate new infection.

Please note that the initial tissue phase of replication is usually a lengthy process measured in weeks or sometimes months. If bites occur on the head or neck, incubation may be much shorter and measured in days. In either case, prompt post-exposure treatment assures greatest protection. Flushing and cleansing wounds is imperative and equally important to the administration of biologics.

### *Diagnosis*

Diagnosis in various animal species can best be accomplished by direct fluorescent antibody stain of brain tissue. Earlier testing methods using dye-stained smears of brain tissue and looking for Negri bodies are less accurate and considered presumptive tests. Other testing methods employing injections of CNS homogenate into suckling mice are cumbersome, expensive, and unnecessary. Fluorescent microscopy techniques are the gold standard for reliable diagnosis. Some reference laboratories offer new molecular testing techniques that allow for identification of strains and comparison of virus-strains at the genetic level.

Usually only the animal's head needs to be submitted for exam, although entire bat carcasses should be submitted to identify species. If possible, do not freeze specimens. Chill the head as soon as possible (cool under running water if ambient temperature is high or animal was freshly euthanized), pack in ice and submit for laboratory testing by the most expedient means available. It is satisfactory to delay any treatment except wound cleansing and care if the test results will be available within one to two days, unless severe bites have occurred in the head or neck region. So injured tissue can be exposed to oxygen, try to leave wounds unsutured.

Human clinical diagnosis may be confirmed by skin biopsy of the neck area to include some hair follicles and corneal impressions or brain biopsy for direct immunofluorescent antibody testing and nucleic acid amplification (e.g. polymerase chain reaction). Collection of saliva, throat swabs or tracheal aspirates may provide virus if collected in the first two weeks of illness. Serological testing of blood serum or cerebral spinal fluid (CSF) may be of limited value beginning after clinical onset but before administration of any rabies biologics. Rabies virus antibody in the CSF, regardless of the rabies immunization history, suggests a rabies virus infection.

The clinical picture prompting a rabies diagnosis is a nonspecific prodromal illness including fever, chills, malaise, fatigue, insomnia, anorexia, headache, anxiety, and irritability. There may be sensory changes at the site of the bite. This is followed by periods of hyperexcitability, confusion, hallucinations, seizures, and occasionally uncontrolled or even aggressive behavior. Aerophobia or apparent dread of air in motion and spasms of the swallowing muscles perceived as fear of water (hydrophobia) may be observed. Attempts to swallow lead to severe, painful, pharyngeal spasms. There is often progression to paralysis, coma, and multiple organ failure, with death usually occurring within 14 days of clinical onset.

### *Post-exposure Treatment and Prevention*

There are only two well-documented cases of human survival from clinical rabies in the medical literature. Both of these patients had some post-exposure treatment. Given these circumstances, it is essential for the reader to understand rabies protection rests on preventing exposure to rabies-associated animal reservoirs by immunizing their companion animals. In any case, if a high-risk exposure does occur (i.e. bite by known or likely rabid animal), administration of globulin and vaccine is essential before the virus enters nerve tissue. Often individuals may not be aware of direct exposure (extensive non-bite saliva contact during work- or recreation-related casual dog contact) or may experience unwitting exposure (bat bite during sleep). Such cases justify need for pre-exposure immunization. Careful assessment of vocations and avocations provide opportunity to identify individuals that would benefit from vaccination (e.g. travelers to rabies endemic areas for visits exceeding four weeks).

Pre-exposure immunization is comprised of three sequential doses of a licensed rabies vaccine (see Table 1) on days 0, 7, and 21 or 28. Day 28 provides better response than day 21. In the U.S.

**TABLE 1. Rabies Biologics—United States, 1999**

| *Human Rabies Vaccine* | *Product Name* | *Manufacturer* |
|---|---|---|
| Human diploid cell vaccine (HDCV) | | Aventis Pasteur |
| • Intramuscular | Imovax Rabies | Phone: (800) VACCINE (822-2463) |
| • Intradermal | Imovax Rabies I.D.* | |
| Rabies vaccine adsorbed (RVA) | Rabies Vaccine Adsorbed (RVA) | BioPort Corporation Phone: (517) 335-8120 |
| • Intramuscular | | |
| Purified chick embryo cell vaccine (PCEC) | RabAvert | Chiron Corporation Phone: (800) CHIRON8 (244-7668) |
| • Intramuscular | | |
| Rabies immune globulin (RIG) | Imogam Rabies-HT | Aventis Pasteur Phone: (800) VACCINE (822-2463) |
| | BayRab | Bayer Corporation Pharmaceutical Div. Phone: (800) 288-8370 |

*Removed from production February 2001.

any of the three licensed vaccines are satisfactory for pre-exposure immunization. The human diploid cell vaccine is also approved for intradermal vaccination utilizing a specific product designed for that use (Imovax ID™) (Table 2). It is important that an individual skilled in *intradermal* vaccination injects this vaccine and that it be injected in the lateral aspect of the *upper arm.* In addition, concurrent administration of oral antimalarial drugs is known to reduce the immunogenicity of this *intradermal* vaccination product. Accordingly antimalarial drugs should be avoided until fully immunized or if necessary to initiate/continue antimalarial drugs, administration of any rabies *intramuscular* product is recommended. Note that all FDA licensed intramuscular rabies

**TABLE 2. Rabies Pre-exposure Prophylaxis Schedule—United States, 1999**

| *Type of Vaccination* | *Route* | *Regimen* |
|---|---|---|
| Primary | Intramuscular | HDCV, PCEC, or RVA; 1.0 mL (deltoid area), one each on days 0*, 7, and 21 or 28 |
| | Intradermal | HDCV; 0.1 mL, one each on days 0*, 7, and 21 or 28 |
| Booster | Intramuscular | HDCV, PCEC, or RVA; 1.0 mL (deltoid area), day 0* only |
| | Intradermal | HDCV, 0.1 mL, day 0* only |

HDCV = human diploid cell vaccine; PCEC = purified chick embryo cell vaccine; RVA = rabies vaccine adsorbed.

* Day 0 is the day the first dose of vaccine is administered.

vaccines are thought to be fully interchangeable but only one product for a series of injections is recommended.

Post-exposure treatment management is essential for all bite wounds or serious non-bite exposures when the animal is known or presumed rabid or the animal's status remains unknown. After a bite, initial treatment should include vigorous washing with soap and flushing of the wound with water. Please view this procedure to be as important and perhaps more important than administration of biologics in the prevention of rabies. (In experimental animals, cleansing of wounds with a 20% soap solution reduced the risk of rabies by 90%.) Next, if at all possible, apprehend and secure the offending animal, taking measures to avoid additional injury. If the animal is a domestic dog or cat, it is recommended to confine the animal for observation whether immunized or not, and monitor for ten days for signs of rabies including excess salivation, aggressive behavior, not eating or drinking, and difficulty walking. If suspect signs develop, the animal should be euthanized and examined immediately for rabies. If the offending animal is a wildlife species, especially a carnivore/

omnivore or bat, it should be immediately euthanized and examined for rabies. If reliable laboratory services are not available, it is appropriate to assume a worst case scenario (i.e. probable rabies exposure) and initiate post-exposure prophylaxis.

If treatment is indicated, the patient's rabies vaccination history comes under consideration. If previously vaccinated, the patient should receive two doses of intramuscular vaccine spaced three days apart (Table 2). *Rabies immune globulin should not be administered and in fact is contraindicated since it can produce immune complexes that affect kidney function.*

If not previously vaccinated, and the patient experienced an exposure justifying treatment, then a full course of vaccine (any of the three intramuscular cell culture vaccines) should be administered IM in the deltoid muscles of the upper arm on days 0, 3, 7, 14 and 28 (Table 3). In addition, on day 0 the patient should receive rabies immune globulin at a dose of 20 IU/kg body weight (2-mL/33.3 lbs. body wt.). Up to the full dose of this product should be injected in the area of the bite if anatomically feasible. The remainder should be injected IM in the gluteal muscle group or upper thigh in small children. Vaccine should not be administered near the site of this globulin injection.

Clearly the patients with pre-exposure vaccination have significant advantages. First, they may be protected against unknown exposures. Second, their post-exposure management is much simpler and lower in cost. With elapsing time there are various protocols to maintain satisfactory immunity. After primary immunization (or even post-exposure immunization), patients with continuing risk of rabies exposure are encouraged to periodically assess their immune titers in lieu of receiving booster vaccine doses. Subsequent doses of vaccine are associated with a 6% rate of immune complex-like reactions including generalized urticaria, sometimes accompanied by arthralgia, arthritis, angioedema, nausea, vomiting, fever, and malaise. None of these reactions have been life-threatening. Optimally, rabies immune titers using the rapid fluorescent focus inhibition test (RFFIT) should

**TABLE 3. Rabies Post-exposure Prophylaxis Schedule. Adapted from Recommendations of the Advisory Committee of Immunization Practices: Human rabies prevention—United States, 1999.**

| *Vaccination Status* | *Treatment* | *Regimen** |
|---|---|---|
| Not previously vaccinated | Wound cleansing | Immediate thorough cleansing of all wounds with soap and water. Irrigate with a virucidal agent such as a povidone-iodine solution. |
| | RIG | Administer 20 IU/kg body weight; no more than the recommended dose should dose should be given. If anatomically feasible, **the full dose** should be infiltrated around the wound(s) and any remaining volume should be administered IM at an anatomical site distant from vaccine administration. |
| | Vaccine | PCEC, RVA, or HDCV 1.0 mL, IM (deltoid area[†]), one each on days 0[‡], 3, 7, 14, and 28. |
| Previously vaccinated[§] | Wound cleansing | Immediate thorough cleansing of all wounds with soap and water. Irrigate with a virucidal agent such as a povidone-iodine solution. |
| | RIG | RIG should **not** be administered. |
| | Vaccine | PCEC, RVA, or HDCV 1.0 mL, IM (deltoid area[†]), one each on days 0[‡], and 3. |

RIG = rabies immune globulin; PCEC = purified chick embryo cell vaccine; RVA = rabies vaccine adsorbed; HDCV = human diploid cell vaccine; IM, intramuscular.

*These regimens are applicable for all age groups, including children.

[†]The deltoid area is the only acceptable site of vaccination for adults and older children. For younger children, the outer aspect of the thigh may be used. Vaccine should never be administered in the gluteal area.

[‡]Day 0 is the day the first dose of vaccine is administered.

[§]Any person with a history of pre-exposure vaccination with PCEC, RVA, or HDCV; prior post-exposure prophylaxis with PCEC, RVA, or HDCV; or previous vaccination with any other type of rabies vaccine and a documented history of antibody response to the prior vaccination.

be checked every two to five years. In the absence of titers and assuming continued high-risk exposures, it would be prudent to receive boosters (either IM or ID) at some frequency in the two to five year range.

Outsiders traveling in areas without up-to-date medical facilities may begin treatment with nerve tissue vaccine or cell culture vaccine. Some developing countries use a purified equine rabies immune globulin (ERIG) for initial passive immunization. The incidence of adverse reactions has been low (0.8%–6.0%), and most of those that occurred were minor. In any case, if exposed outsiders cannot access treatment used in their home country, they are encouraged to use WHO approved treatment. Then when they return to their home countries after initiation of post-exposure treatment, it may be necessary to provide additional therapy.

### *Rabies Control*

Rabies control can be achieved by immunizing our domestic animals, especially companion animals which should include horses and registered or valuable livestock that is handled or exhibited a great deal. In this instance it is very true that "vaccine in bottles does no good." As a minimum, companion animals should be immunized if resources permit, recognizing that sometimes dogs are not associated with any given household. Experience in Philippines and Ecuador have shown that depopulation of dogs is not practical and often leads to social disruption of dog populations that may lead to increased rabies transmission.

Horses and livestock may also be immunized but cost for the procedure may have to be balanced against available resources. There clearly are incentives to vaccinate animals if the carnivore reservoir is the main source of exposure. Insectivorous bats are problematic in that they do not figure prominently in transmission to terrestrial animals but do pose appreciable risk to humans. Accordingly, it is important to eliminate bats from homes and buildings. It is also wise to encourage would-be "spelunkers" to be pre-immunized and don protective clothing/gear before entering bat caves and harborages. If hematophagus bats are the main source of rabies, there is no immunization technology (i.e. oral vaccine) for addressing this reservoir. The capture of these bats from their colonies, spreading anticoagulant chemicals on their backs and releasing them is used in Latin American countries, especially in known rabies infected colonies. The bats ingest the anticoagulants in mutual grooming, leading to depopulation of these colonies. The most common approach is by vaccinating cattle in infected bat areas thereby protecting this most bat-attacked species.

Given these dismal observations, the fact remains that as a minimum, U.S. workers and volunteers overseas in rabies endemic countries should receive pre-exposure immunization for rabies. In the immunological sense it provides a coat of armor against a 100% fatal disease.

Outside workers and volunteers in rabies endemic areas of the world should receive pre-exposure immunization for rabies.

CHAPTER 2

# Tuberculosis in Animals and Humans

*By Dr. Mitchell Esse*

### *Bovine Tuberculosis in Animals and Human Beings*

### *The Mycobacteria*

Tuberculosis is an infectious, contagious disease of animals and human beings. It is caused by three bacterial species of the genus Mycobacterium. Mycobacterium tuberculosis is infectious to all mammalian species, including humans, and to several avian species, giving it the greatest host range of all of the pathogenic mycobacteria. *M.tuberculosis* primarily affects humans but can also be transmitted to non-human primates, swine, dogs, cats, elephants and other exotic species, as well as parrots. *M.avium* causes progressive, usually fatal tuberculosis in most avian species, and is infectious to swine, cattle, and many other mammalian species in which it usually causes limited, non-progressive disease. Humans are also susceptible to *M.avium* infection, but are very resistant to the disease.

The pathogenic mycobacteria are in the genus of the family *Mycobacteriaceae,* containing slender, aerobic, Gram positive, rod shaped acid fast bacilli. Acid fast denotes bacteria that when stained with aniline dyes are not decolorized by mineral acids. They are slow growers and do not reproduce outside the host except fastidiously on artificial media where weeks may pass before the appearance of visible colonies. They are long lived in moist, cool environments and are very resistant to disinfectants. Mycobacteria are readily destroyed by direct sunlight or heat 160°F or greater.

## HISTORY

*M.bovis* had been causing TB in the animal kingdom long before invading humanity. However, after the domestication of cattle between 8000–4000 BC, there is evidence of human infection by *M.bovis*, likely through milk ingestion. This coincides with archaeological evidence of spinal TB (Potts disease) 5000–1000 BC. *M.bovis* was the likely pathogen in human TB until 1000 BC. After 1000 BC, widespread pulmonary TB emerged. In fact, *M.tuberculosis* probably is an evolved, specialized form of *M.bovis* developed among milk-drinking Indo-Europeans who then spread the disease during their migration into western Europe and Eurasia. By the 1st millennium BC, *M.tuberculosis* causing pulmonary TB had spread through the known world. The earliest tangible record of pulmonary TB dates between 668–626 BC and was contained in the library of the Assyrian King Assanbanipal. The classic TB signs (cough, expectoration, hemoptysis, wasting of the body) were well recognized. Exact pathological and anatomical descriptions of the disease began to appear in the seventeenth century. In his Opera Medica of 1679, Sylvius was the first to identify actual tubercles as a consistent and characteristic change in the lungs and other areas of consumptive patients. He also described their progression to abscesses and cavities. Manget described the pathological features of miliary tuberculosis in 1702. The earliest references to the infectious nature of the disease appear in seventeenth century Italian medical literature. An edict issued by the Republic of Lucca in 1699 states that "henceforth, human health should no longer be endangered by objects remaining after the death of a consumptive. The names of the deceased should be reported to the authorities, and measures undertaken for disinfection." In 1720, the English physician Benjamin Marten was the first to conjecture in his publication, *A New Theory of Consumption,* that TB could be caused by "wonderfully minute living creatures," which, once they had gained a foothold in the body, could generate the lesions and symptoms of the disease.

During the 1800's and early 1900's, tuberculosis was the most prevalent infectious disease of cattle and swine in the United States, causing more losses among farm animals than all other infectious diseases combined. In 1882, Dr. Robert Koch, an Austrian physician, reported in his paper, *The Etiology of Tuberculosis,* his discovery of the cause of tuberculosis in humans, cattle, and other animal species. He called this bacterium the "tubercle bacillus." Only 10 years later, Dr. Koch reported his discovery of tuberculin, making possible the diagnosis of tuberculosis in humans and animals before the onset of clinical signs or death from the disease. Along with Russia and Denmark, the U.S. perceived almost immediately, the potential of tuberculin for controlling, then eliminating the disease from the bovine species. Just one year following Dr. Koch's announcement, a small supply of tuberculin was given to Dr. L. Pearson, University of Pennsylvania. Thus began university centered efforts against tuberculosis, which resulted in small tuberculosis-free areas surrounded by wide spans of tuberculosis affected herds. These tuberculosis-free areas soon dissolved as cattle movements went on as usual. The District of Columbia became the first political entity to undertake tuberculosis control procedures, where in 1909 the prevalence in cattle was 18.9%. By 1911, the prevalence was reduced to 1.37%, and by 1925, to 0.00, making DC the first defined area of the world to achieve the total eradication of bovine tuberculosis. From these early experiences emerge two important considerations for dealing with tuberculosis in livestock. We learned the tuberculin test accurately detected infected individuals in time to permit their removal from the herd before they could spread the bacillus to other animals, making it possible to free a herd from disease.

Without effective movement control, any testing program would not only fail to free an area of disease, but would instead actually increase the rate of area spread, by owners selectively culling test positive animals which then enter trade channels. Thus formed the origins of the bovine tuberculosis eradication concept.

Information in the Animal Health yearbook of the Food of Agriculture Organization-World Health Organization (1995) indicates that bovine tuberculosis occurs worldwide wherever cattle are found.

### *The Disease*

Lesions of tuberculosis result from the host's immunological attempts to destroy and seal off the infecting mycobacteria. This process results in the formation of nodules, called tubercles from which the disease gets its name. Tubercles form in grape like clusters, which eventually merge together forming abscesses which displace normal tissues with caseous, often granular necrotic material. Tuberculosis lesions may be found in any organ or body cavity. In early stages of the disease these lesions are difficult to find, but in later stages the lesions of bovine tuberculosis become very evident, most commonly in the lungs and associated lymph nodes, and in the lymph nodes of the head and intestinal tract. Lesions may also occur in the abdominal organs, reproductive organs, nervous system, joints, and bones. *M.bovis* tuberculosis usually takes many months to develop, and in most cases results in a chronic, progressive disease of long standing. The disease may be fulminating at times, and cause death of the host within a few weeks. Most often, however, the organism will lie dormant within the host's body for years, causing progressive disease only with the onset of old age, or other circumstance associated with reduced immunity. Cattle, bison, deer, and elk with bovine tuberculosis often show few or no clinical signs and appear to be in prime condition, yet may show extensive disease on slaughter inspection. Once symptoms appear, the animal's condition rapidly deteriorates and death ensues.

Bovine type tuberculosis in humans, as in most mammalian species, is primarily a pulmonary disease. In human beings, pulmonary tuberculosis caused by *M.bovis* is pathologically and clinically indistinguishable from that caused by *M.tuberculosis. M.bovis,* however, has a greater predilection than *M.tuberculosis* for infecting extra pulmonary sites, such as bone, the joints, the inner ear, the spinal column and intervertebral spaces from which it readily spreads to the meninges and brain. This makes *M.bovis* infection particularly difficult to treat because at these sites blood circulation is hardly capable of delivering antimycobacterial drugs at therapeutic levels.

Historically, pre-eradication, pre-pasteurization, the primary target of *M.bovis* infection was the very young who consumed raw mild from tuberculous cows. Abdominal tuberculosis caused by *M.bovis* was common in children who often died from peritonitis resulting from a perforated tuberculous gut. Pulmonary tuberculosis is more readily acquired by close association with infected animals, such as by workers in infected dairy herds, and by abattoir workers inhaling infectious aerosols generated during slaughter of tuberculous animals and cleanup. Scoliosis (crooked spine, hunchback) resulting from tuberculous disintegrations of the vertebrae was a common complication seen with *M.bovis* infection. Scrofula, characterized by enlarged, abscessed, draining tuberculous lymph nodes of the neck, is the most common clinical disease associated with infectious raw milk consumption. Clinical scrofula caused by *M.bovis* is virtually eradicated where milk pasteurization is required by regulation.

### *Tuberculosis Transmission*

Bovine tuberculosis is primarily a pulmonary disease. It is estimated that 90% of spread is by the respiratory route. Invisible droplets (aerosols) carrying tubercle bacilli may be expelled by exhalation or coughing of infected animals, then inhaled by susceptible animals or humans. The risk of exposure is greatest in enclosed areas such as barns and in feeding and watering areas where animals may concentrate for long periods. Inhalation or aerosols is the most common route of infection for farm and ranch workers and veterinarians who work with diseased livestock. Bovine tuberculosis can be transmitted from animals to humans and vice versa, the most common means of transmission being the respiratory route. In the Nordic countries, Sweden, Finland and Denmark, in which bovine tuberculosis was successfully eradicated decades ago, new found infection in their cattle herds is regularly traced to *M.bovis* infected humans. Senior family members exposed to tuberculous cattle in their youth (1930's and 1940's) develop progressive disease in their old age and transmit disease to herds now owned by their grandchildren. Young animals and humans can contract the disease by drinking raw milk from infected cows. Calves, swine and other livestock species are readily infected by nursing on their infected dams.

Early in this century bovine type tuberculosis was widespread in humans consuming unpasteurized milk from the marketplace. With the advent of meat inspection, the risk is negligible of acquiring tuberculosis from consuming meat and meat products. The original meat inspection procedure was designed primarily to detect tuberculosis, a fact that has not appreciably changed today. Bovine tuberculosis in wildlife can be spread and perpetuated by wild carnivora or omnivores consuming tuberculosis from ingesting infected carcass parts at rendering establishments. Skin tuberculosis, and tuberculous puncture wounds and cuts were common in abattoir workers, veterinarians and pathologists. Tuberculosis can be transmitted congenitally; approximately one percent of calves of tuberculosis dams are born with tuberculosis.

### *Diagnosis*

Tuberculous humans and animals develop an immune response which can be elicited by the tuberculin skin test. Tuberculin is a sterile diagnostic reagent made by growing *M.bovis*, Strain AN5 Bacilli on culture media, sterilizing with heat, and removing all particulate matter by filtration. The protein components are then precipitated out of the culture filtrate making purified protein derivative (PPD). Bovine PPD intradermal tuberculin is made by reconstituting such tuberculoprotein to 1.0 mg per mL. The dose is 0.1 mL (5000 tuberculin units) injected intradermally in cattle, bison, deer, elk and most other domestic livestock. The injection site is examined by palpation about 72 hours post-injection for the appearance of a characteristic response which would indicate previous exposure to a pathogenic mycobacterium. Further diagnostic methods are necessary to confirm the presence of tuberculosis.

In humans, these tests include chest x-rays and sputum cultures. For animals, the comparative cervical tuberculin test (CCT) is used to determine the likelihood of *M.bovis* being the causal agent of the reaction. The CCT utilizes paired injections of biologically balanced tuberculins, PPD Bovine and PPD Avium, to which animals infected with *M.bovis* will respond preferentially to the bovine tuberculin. Some or all of the following methods can be used in diagnosis: serological tests, whole blood tests for lymphocyte stimulation and/or gamma interferon production, genetic analysis and culture of mycobacteria recovered in life, post mortem examination, histopathology and culture. Advanced diagnostic procedures become increasingly important as nations deal more comprehensively with alternate livestock species, with farmed deer and elk, and with tuberculosis in zoos, including rare and endangered species.

### *Recent Advances of Diagnosis of Bovine Tuberculosis*

Until recently the only practical and reasonably reliable diagnostic test was the tuberculin test which has had problems with sensitivity and specificity. It has several other drawbacks in that it requires handling animals twice: once for the injection and again to check for a reaction at the injection site. This is often a problem in beef animals that are not used to being handled.

Further, the skin test interferes with the immune state of the animal so that it cannot be re-tested for minimum of 60 days.

In the past few years, the Australian government at its CSIRO and CSL facilities, have developed a blood test which can be run overnight. If an animal or human has been exposed to TB, the T cells in the blood will produce gamma interferon (IFN-y); a simple test is then used to detect the presence of the IFS-y.

The test is approved for use in Australia, New Zealand and Romania and approval is pending in several other countries, with major trials being conducted in many other areas. It is more expensive than the tuberculin test but that is offset in most cases by not having to handle the cattle twice. A companion test for use in humans is approved in Australia and New Zealand with trials being undertaken in other countries.

Another recent advance in diagnosis of TB is a new test developed at The National Animal Disease Center in the USA. It uses a polymerase chain reaction (PCR) technique. It can be conducted in 3 days versus the current culture methods, which can take up to 3 months. Besides greatly shortening the time for diagnosis, it is very specific for *M.bovis* and eliminates other mycobacteria.

### *Control and Eradication Programs*

Many factors affect the implementation of control and eradication programs for tuberculosis around the world. Economics, traditions, location of the animals, availability of trained personnel and many other factors affect the stage of programs in different areas and countries. In almost every country there has been some degree of activity undertaken toward the control of the disease.

### *Other Factors and Thoughts in Controlling Tuberculosis in Animals and its Spread to Humans*

A. Summary of Successful Control Efforts:

1. On-farm testing of cattle, and removal of positive animals is the basis of control programs. The editor will be glad to provide

readers with details of on-farm control measures that have been successful. The details are too lengthy for this publication.

2. Commercial pasteurization of milk and milk products, especially around large cities. Home pasteurization of milk and milk products. An irony is that many in the past boiled milk to preserve it. This was probably a factor in lowering the incidence of tuberculosis in humans. However, when refrigeration became available many stopped boiling milk, a change that may cause a rise in the rate of infection.
3. Meat inspection has definitely been a major factor in removing much of the infected meat products that would otherwise be consumed by humans.
4. At some stage of a control program, it will be necessary to trace positive animals back to their premise of origin as closely as possible to locate other herds and areas that might have tuberculosis. In addition, suspect animals at slaughter should also be traced back to their premise of origin, if possible, in order to locate possible infected herds and areas. The sooner trace backs from farms with positive animals and from slaughter plants is done, the more efficient a control program will be.
5. Restrictions on movement of animals between untested herds and areas into tested herds and areas. While this is usually done in later stages of a control program, it would pay big dividends any time it can be implemented.

B. Other Factors in Preventing the Spread of the Disease:

1. Cook all meat for human consumption well done with special attention to large bones which can be difficult to cook.
2. Thorough cooking of garbage intended for animals. Slaughter house waste and waste food from hospitals should receive special attention. In many areas the incidence of *M. bovis* in pigs is almost as frequent as it is in cattle. Cooking garbage being fed to pigs could greatly lessen the spread of tuberculosis.
3. Tuberculosis testing of humans working with dairy animals. In the past there have been incidents in which humans and cattle both had tuberculosis. When tuberculosis was controlled in the dairy herd, the animals later contracted the disease from older humans.
4. Do not feed raw milk to pigs. In many areas this is a primary means of spread. It is not uncommon to feed milk to pigs, especially where transportation of milk to market is a problem.

5. Emaciated older animals, especially those with enlarged lymph nodes and coughing, should be removed from the herd since they are highly suspicious of tuberculosis. This would be especially true if there was a history of the disease in the herd.

C. Final thought: With the increasing interest in control of brucellosis and the fact of tuberculosis also being a major problem, it might be well to consider combining the two programs when possible.

### *Acknowledgments*

Dr. Jerome Harms, University of Wisconsin, USA for historical information Bacteriology Lecture Topics: Tuberculosis. Mr. Niall Byrne, Science consultant, Byrne Young Communication, P.O. Box 199, Drysdale 3222 Australia for information on the blood tests developed in Australia for diagnosis of TB. Dr. Ray Hines of the Clemson University Animal Diagnostic Laboratory in Columbia, SC, USA for resource material and suggestions for completing this paper.

CHAPTER 3

# Brucellosis in Animals and Humans

*By Dr. David Warner*

## BRUCELLOSIS—HISTORY AND REVIEW

Brucellosis is a reproductive disease of animals caused by gram negative facultative intracellular bacteria of the genus *Brucella.* The disease is zoonotic and is often referred to as "undulant fever" in humans. Due to the costs of reproductive inefficiencies of animals and the debilitating disease in humans, agricultural officials in many countries have determined to control or eradicate the disease in domestic livestock.

Much of the early modern work with brucellosis took place in the Middle East before the turn of the 20th century. *Brucella melitensis* was cultured from human patients at a British military infirmary on the island of Malta by Bruce in 1887. Brucellosis was epidemic among the soldiers as well as civilians on the island. Epidemiologic studies conducted under Bruce in 1907 demonstrated goats as reservoir, and untreated milk as a vehicle of infection. *Brucella melitensis* is thought to have been introduced to the Americas by Spanish conquistadors with infected goats.

Distribution of brucellosis is nearly world wide, with the exception of a few countries that have undertaken aggressive eradication campaigns. In North America, Canada has eradicated the disease, and the United States had no infected cattle herds at the end of the year 2000.

### *Brucellosis in Humans*

Despite the ready availability and the relative low cost of effective antimicrobial therapy, brucellosis remains a leading bacterial zoonosis worldwide. Like the resurgence of tuberculosis in the United States in the 1980's, brucellosis roared back into world prominence, especially in the Middle East. In the 1990's, the Balkans and the other former Soviet countries were troubled with increasing human and animal brucellosis outbreaks. Although brucellosis is rarely a killer, the disease is extremely debilitating, and often misdiagnosed. The sequelae of untreated brucellosis may result in permanent disability.

The onset of clinical disease in humans usually falls between three days and two weeks post-exposure. The signs are nondescript, including fever, malaise, and myalgia, and are often diagnosed as a "flu virus." The fever and accompanying signs often abate after several days, only to return days later, with equal or greater severity. Recurrences are quite common in the absence of treatment, and sequelae may include arthritis (usually spinal), moderate to severe mental illness (usually depression), orchitis (especially *B suis*), or other disorders depending on the end organ in which the brucella localizes. Repeated exposures to brucella have been reported to cause allergic skin reactions locally, or painful firm lesions resulting from a delayed hypersensitivity reaction. These types of reactions are most commonly reported in veterinarians.

Brucellosis in humans is either a food borne disease or an occupational disease. It is acquired through consumption of unpasteurized milk or milk products. Soft cheeses made from unpasteurized milk are common vehicles of infection. Occupational exposures include farmers, veterinarians, abattoir workers, hunters, and laboratory workers. Farmers and veterinarians are most often exposed while assisting dystocia or cleaning afterbirth of affected animals. Use of live vaccines, e.g., Strain 19 or RB 51, is another means by which veterinarians contract brucellosis. Needle sticks and ocular exposure are the most common vaccine accidents. Abattoir workers and hunters may become infected by contact with blood from *B. suis* infected swine. Laboratory exposures usually result from aerosols generated by improper centrifugation, mouth pipetting, or other careless behaviors.

The brucellae to which humans are susceptible are *B. melitensis, B. suis,* and *B. abortus* (Strain 19 is a modified *B. abortus*), in order of pathogenicity. In general, the rough colonial brucellae are not pathogenic to man, including *B. ovis* and *B. canis.* Rough brucella 51, the vaccine strain, is intermediate in pathogenicity to humans, occasionally causing symptoms with infection.

Prevention of brucellosis in humans is accomplished by pasteurization of milk, which may be accomplished at home by heating milk to 60° C for 30 minutes. Boiling temperature is 100° C. Occupational exposure to vaccine is minimized when vaccination is conducted or supervised by a veterinarian. Protective eyewear, rubber gloves or sleeves, and other protective gear may reduce human exposure to brucellosis when handling infected fetuses, afterbirth, or when butchering infected hogs.

Treatment of brucellosis calls for lengthy tetracycline therapy. The drug of choice is doxycycline, 100 mg, twice a day for three to four weeks. Recurrences are rare if the entire treatment regimen is followed.

### *Epidemiology of Brucellosis in Animals*

Brucellosis is a reproductive disease, characterized by symptoms in males and females alike. Affected males variably show orchitis, epididymitis, infertility, and sterility. Affected females of all species may show infertility; however, abortion is common in cows, nannies, bitches, and sows. *B. suis, B. ovis,* and *B. canis* are easily spread during breeding, while *B. abortus* and *B. melitensis* are not. The bull or billy may occasionally contract infection during breeding, and therefore may serve as sentinel animals in heavily infected herds.

The primary route of transmission of *B. abortus* and *B. melitensis* is by oral contact with heavily contaminated placental and fetal material after abortion or birth. In close quarters, the organism may enter via the conjunctiva. Control measures should take account of the mode of transmission and times of highest exposure of the herd.

Transmission rate of brucellosis in herds is most dependent on two variables: host resistance and exposure level of the organism. Host resistance is determined by innate genetic factors and acquired resistance through exposure to vaccine or natural infection. Vaccination is the most practical means to boost herd resistance, and is commonly used in control programs. Genes that determine resistance to brucellosis have been identified in cattle and, in the future, breeding programs may be employed to confer innate herd resistance. Exposure to natural infection has also been observed to provide herd resistance, however, the disadvantages are obvious. After the initial abortion storm in affected herds, the live birth rate returns close to normal, and the herd appears asymptomatic except that some heifers will abort.

Exposure level to brucella is determined by the shedding rate in affected animals, survival of organisms in the environment, and animal density in the herd. The shedding rate of affected animals is influenced by innate and acquired resistance, i.e., vaccinated or naturally resistant animals tend to shed at a much lower rate, and animals that have aborted tend to shed fewer organisms at subsequent calvings. Survival of brucella in the contaminated placenta is favored by cool temperatures and moisture in the environment. High ambient temperature, sunlight, and desiccation limit survival of brucella to a matter of days. Environmental conditions should be considered when restocking contaminated pastures. Cleaning and disinfection should be employed in cool, sheltered locations like barns and sheds. Brucella is susceptible to any of the antibacterial disinfectants including sodium hypochlorite (bleach), sodium hydroxide, Nolvasan, One Stroke, etc. Probability of exposure is increased by high stocking density on pastures, confinement rearing, or other management practices that concentrate animals into a small area, e.g., supplemental winter feeding. It is no wonder that brucellosis transmission in North American dairies can be a nightmare, based on management practices that concentrate high risk animals at the time of calving!

Even though the *Brucella* species are relatively host specific, interspecies transmission does occur. *Brucella melitensis* is known to transmit from goats to cattle, and cases of spread among cattle have been reported. *Brucella abortus* may be spread to cattle by infected bitches at whelping. Likewise, transmission of *B. abortus* from bison and elk to cattle may occur in heavily infected, highly concentrated populations like those of the Greater Yellowstone Park area in the United States. Equidae are dead end hosts for *B. abortus*, however there are numerous examples of fistulous withers horses spreading brucellosis to cattle. An interesting example of interspecies transmission complicating diagnosis in the final stage of brucellosis eradication in the United States is transmission of *B. suis* from feral swine to cattle in the Gulf Coast states. Fortunately, *B. suis* has not been shown to spread among cattle.

*Brucella abortus* and *B. melitensis* are community diseases, and effective management dictates that the entire community be included in control measures. The factors most responsible for interherd transmission of the disease include acquisition of replacement animals and physical proximity to infected herds. Communities tend to establish accepted practices of replacement animal acquisition, whether by sharing, trading or purchasing. For prevention efforts the frequency and source of replacement animals must be determined. Brucellosis does not observe a fence line as a boundary; in fact, fence line contact herds are at highest risk of becoming infected. Another community factor to consider is mechanical vectors such as dogs and other scavengers that can drag contaminated fetuses across property lines.

### *Diagnosis of Brucellosis*

The diagnosis of brucellosis in humans and animals is established by history of exposure, clinical signs, serologic tests, and bacterial culture. Exposure history and an agglutination of ELISA test are usually sufficient for diagnosis in humans. Occasionally, an agglutination test that eliminates IgM antibody will be employed to rule out old resolved infection or cross reactions to closely related bacteria.

Diagnosis in animals is a bit more complicated, because the entire herd must be considered, and serological cross reactions are more prevalent. Use of certain vaccines, e.g. Strain 19, complicate diagnosis in individual animals in the herd. Whole herd serologic testing is recommended for *B. melitensis, B. abortus, B. suis,* and *B. ovis.* A sensitive presumptive test, such as the Card Test of ELISA is first conducted on samples from the entire herd. Individuals positive to this screening test are then subjected to supplemental tests, which have a higher predictive value for infection. If infection is suspected, milk or lymph nodes can be collected for culture to confirm diagnosis. An experienced epidemiologist should be able to make most diagnoses without culture; however a culture positive animal may instill farmer confidence in the diagnostician.

A *Brucella suis* diagnosis is more challenging, because there are no serologic tests with sufficient predictive value for individual animals. Because of this, test and slaughter has been largely abandoned by the United States in favor of herd depopulation.

Because of favorable cross reactivity, tests using *B. abortus* antigen will work effectively for *B. abortus, B. suis,* and *B. melitensis* testing. All commonly used agglutination tests, complement fixation, and ELISA tests used in the United States brucellosis eradication program use a *B. abortus* antigen. *B. abortus* antigen does not work for diagnosis of *B. canis* or *B. ovis*. *Brucella canis* diagnosis using conventional serology is difficult because of false positive reactions, nevertheless, a modified mercaptoethanol agglutination test is the standard for veterinary practice in the United States. *B. ovis* is diagnosed serologically with gel diffusion, complement fixation, and ELISA tests using *B. ovis* antigen. There are some difficulties with *B. ovis* diagnosis in cases where *B. melitensis* is also present, caused by cross reaction.

### *Brucellosis Control and Eradication*

Because brucellosis is an intracellular bacterial infection, treatment of livestock with antimicrobials is neither economical nor effective, as a general rule. Management of the disease generally involves three components:

- Raising herd resistance with vaccine
- Testing and culling reactor animals
- Managing the reproductive cycle

Although not every herd can incorporate all three elements of control, herd cleanup is most effective when the three are used together.

### *Vaccination*

Although numerous vaccines have been used in cattle, sheep, and goats over the years, *B. abortus* Strain 19 and *B. melitensis* Rev. 1 have found widest usage. Rev. 1 is used for prevention of ram epididymitis as well as *B. melitensis* infections. Since 1996, RB 51 has been employed in the final stages of brucellosis eradication in the United States. Vaccines have not traditionally been employed for *B. canis* and *B. suis,* however RB 51 Has been tested in Argentina and the United States in limited trials with swine. A rough *B. suis* vaccine similar to RB 51 is under development for use in swine.

Using vaccines effectively in a control program calls for vaccination of the entire herd, or all herds at risk in the community.

This can be accomplished slowly by calfhood vaccinating replacement animals, or all at once by adult vaccination. In areas where restriction of animal movement or quarantine are not feasible for disease control, revaccination may be necessary. The advent of RB 51 vaccine obviates the persistent post-vaccinal titers that complicate diagnosis when adult vaccinating with Strain 19; therefore, vaccination of the entire herd or community with RB 51 vaccine is recommended.

The fact that effective Brucella vaccines are modified live products introduces some difficulties to control efforts. If proper veterinary administration or supervision is not provided, results of vaccination will likely be disappointing. A viable dose of organisms is required to initiate the cell mediated immune response necessary to protect against Brucella field-strain infection. There is virtually no protection conferred by vaccination with nonviable vaccine. Adult vaccination calls for additional dilution to reduce pathogenicity and post-vaccinal titers. The resulting vaccine is less stable, and must be used within 30 minutes of dilution. The diluted vaccine should also be maintained on ice to insure viability. As mentioned earlier, public health concerns also dictate veterinary supervision of Brucella vaccines.

### *Testing and Culling Reactors*

Periodic whole herd or community testing and removal of reactors is highly recommended to speed the eradication process. Even though Brucella shedding is reduced in a vaccinated population, the source of exposure is not eliminated unless the reactors are removed. A test before calving ensures the removal of most animals incubating the disease before there is opportunity for these animals to expose other animals in the herd.

When a control or eradication effort is started, the area under the program should undertake precautions against continual reintroduction of the disease to the area. If this cannot be accomplished, an otherwise effective program will lose credibility with the farmers. Animals moved into the program area should originate from herds tested negative for brucellosis. Another test should be conducted at the destination farm 30 or more days after arrival. Pregnant animals should remain isolated from the receiving herd until they test negative.

In an aggressive program, animals may be tested by a simple agglutination test like the Card Test at the time they are gathered to vaccinate, and reactors removed at that time. This is practical only in a previously unvaccinated population, due to possible retained vaccination titers. Post-vaccination testing should continue one year past the last removal of reactors, since the incubation period may extend for an entire gestation period. Less aggressive programs call for a minimum of annual testing until two negative annual tests are achieved. Where possible, testing before calving is preferred as long as infection persists in the herd or community.

### *Managing the Reproductive Cycle*

The third element of an effective brucellosis control scheme is management of the reproductive cycle. After all, the reproductive cycle defines the time of high risk for shedding bacteria and resultant exposure to the organism. Two strategies may be employed, and neither one is always practical.

—Limiting the duration of herd exposure to the bull will concentrate the dangerous calving period, reducing the frequency of necessary testing and removal of reactors.

—Segregation of animals by stage of gestation will also reduce the number of animals exposed during the calving period.

### *Other Factors in Brucellosis Eradication*

Since brucellosis is a community disease, the importance of vaccination and testing of all herds concurrently cannot be overemphasized. Movement of infected animals into vaccinated or brucellosis negative herds can renew the cycle of disease in these herds, if not detected and removed. Local and national economic political events can radically alter disease control programs, as witnessed in a handful of Central and South American countries in the past two decades. International boundaries may become meaningless when there is heavy demand for breeding stock, potentially jeopardizing disease control programs. Importers of breeding stock must be careful to identify disease-free stock, or risk losing progress made in disease control efforts. Interstate movement of diseased stock in the United States set back brucellosis eradication numerous times over the last 30 years.

An important part of a national eradication program includes a surveillance component to determine the level of infection in the general population. This often involves testing animals presented for sale or slaughter. Surveillance can help program managers identify infected communities, rank program priorities, and determine progress of the program, since resources are usually limited.

In an eradication program with limited resources, the following elements are minimum requirements:

—Ongoing surveillance
—Complete vaccination of infected communities
—Annual complete test of vaccinated communities until two negative tests are accomplished

If the aim of the program is control instead of eradication, testing can be reduced, but farmer and veterinary education and vaccination must be continued indefinitely. Public health concerns also remain a priority if control is the goal. Public health education regarding pasteurization, safe slaughter and butchering, and vaccination safety should be emphasized.

CHAPTER 4

# African Trypanosomes in Animals and Humans

*By Dr. David S. Peterson*

## HISTORY AND REVIEW

Trypanosomes are elongated, spindle-shaped protozoan parasites of the order Kinetoplastida. Organisms within this order include species that parasitize hosts from plants to humans. Parasites of the genus *Trypanosoma* infect virtually all vertebrates, usually living in the blood and tissue fluids (the American *Trypanosome, T. cruzi,* is an exception, being an intracellular parasite in its vertebrate host.)

African trypanosomiasis is one of the most devastating parasitic diseases, due to the high toll exacted on both human and animal health. *Trypanosoma brucei* was first described in 1895 by Surgeon-Captain David Bruce of the British Army Medical service. Bruce implicated it as the cause of "Tsetse fly disease," known to the Zulu as "loss of spirit" ("nagana" in the Zulu language).

This review will focus on *T. brucei* and *T. congolense,* the causative agents of nagana in domestic ruminants. Both of these organisms are transmitted by biting flies of the genus *Glossina,* otherwise known as the Tsetse fly. Trypanosomes are polymorphic, having different forms in the mammalian and arthropod hosts. As depicted in Figure 1, the infection of the mammalian host is initiated by metacyclic trypanosomes injected with the saliva of the

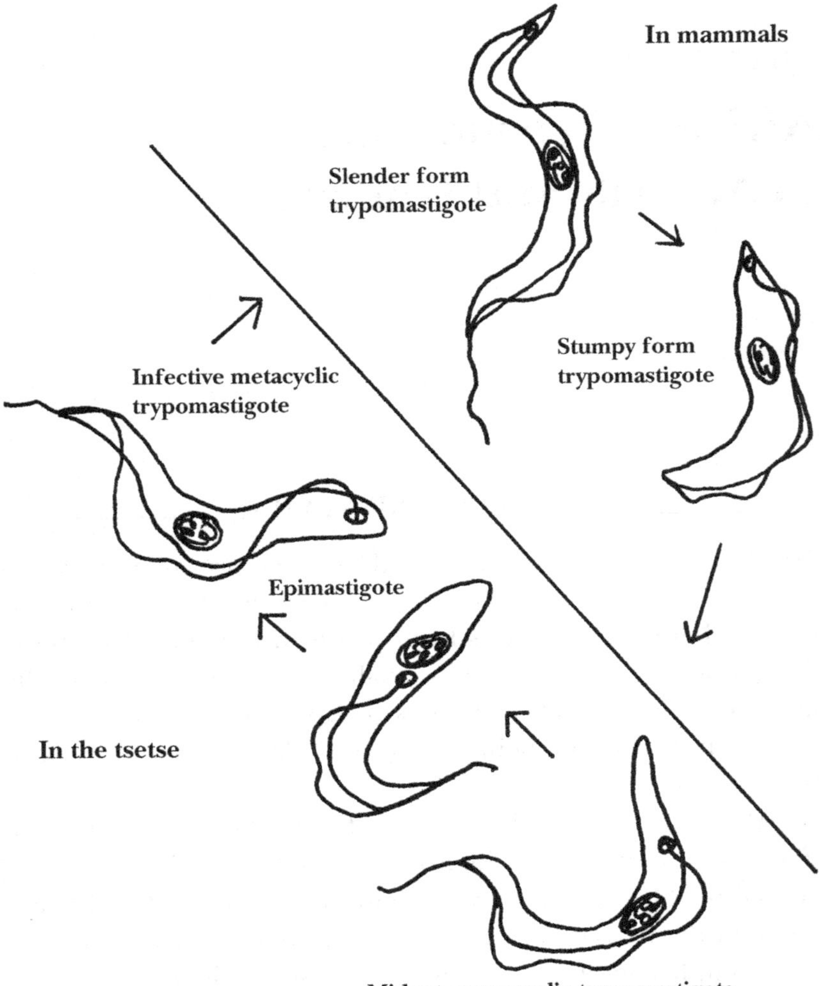


***FIGURE 1.*** **Life cycle of *Trypanosoma brucei*. Distinct morphological forms are seen in the mammalian host and the Tsetse fly.**

tsetse at the beginning of the blood meal. The non-dividing metacyclic trypanosomes soon transform to the long slender blood stream form trypomastigotes. In *T. brucei* a second bloodstream form has been noted; the "short-stumpy" form. It is believed that the latter form is the one actually infectious to the

Tsetse. The short-stumpy form is not seen in infections with *T. congolense*, suggesting that in this species the long-slender form is fully infectious for the insect vector.

Trypanosomes ingested by a Tsetse fly during a blood meal transform to midgut, or procyclic trypanosomes that multiply within the midgut for about 10 days. At this time the parasites migrate forward, eventually reaching the salivary glands. Within the salivary glands another transformation takes place, resulting in the epimastigote, a dividing but non-infective form. After several more rounds of asexual division a final transformation ensues, producing the non-dividing but infective metacyclic trypomastigote.

### *Epidemiology*

The distribution of the Tsetse fly in Africa coincides with those areas endemic for trypanosomiasis and consists of approximately 10 million square kilometers. Figure 2 shows the range of the tsetse covers much of sub-Saharan Africa. Note that transmission does vary over this vast region, and endemicity will be lower in some areas than others. Although the tsetse remain infected for life (up to 11 months), generally the infection rate is low; 2–4%. For comparison, the dotted line indicates the relative size of the continental United States. Imagine if cattle production across the entire U.S. was precluded due to trypanosomiasis! The magnitude of this problem is truly staggering.

### *Pathogenesis*

The clinical course of the disease depends upon the innate susceptibility of the host species. In general the disease takes a more rapid course in animals other than cattle (horses, mules, smaller ruminants and dogs) with death in as little as 15 days. In cattle a chronic condition can develop that lasts several months, however if untreated this usually ends in the death of the host. Anemia is an important feature of the disease and is hemolytic in

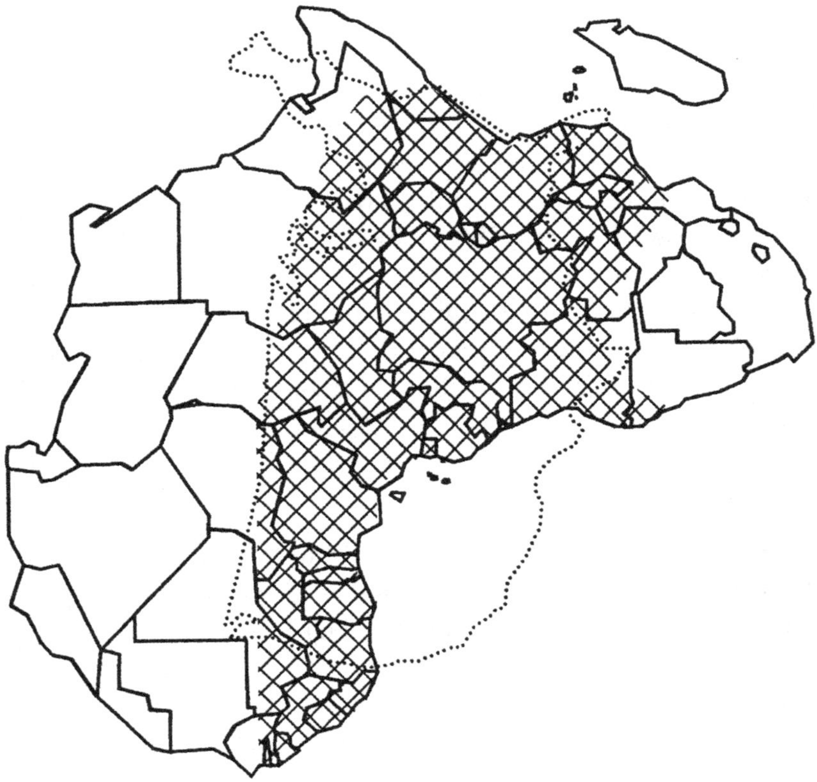

*FIGURE 2.* **Range of the Tsetse fly. The cross hatch pattern denotes those areas of Africa which are home to the tsetse, as well as the trypanosome. For comparison an outline of the continental United States is overlaid on this vast region.**

nature. It has been suggested that parasite antigens released into the circulation may bind to red cells, prompting their removal by the phagocytic system. Enlarged lymph nodes and splenomegaly seem associated with plasma cell hyperplasia and hypergammaglobinemia. In chronic infections the lymphoid organs and spleen may eventually shrink due to overstimulation by parasite antigens leading to tissue exhaustion.

### *Diagnosis*

Clinical findings consistent with nagana in ruminants include anemia, generalized enlargement of the superficial lymph nodes, lethargy and a progressive loss of condition. Peaks of parasitemia are associated with fever and inappetence. Additional observations that are suggestive of trypanosomiasis include reduced weight gain in young animals, and decreased fertility in adults. Infected cows may spontaneously abort, or if carried to term, newborn calves may be small and weak.

Confirmation of a diagnosis of trypanosomiasis requires the demonstration of trypanosomes in blood, bone marrow or cerebral spinal fluid. For blood, both thick and thin smears are prepared. The thick smears offer the best chance of detecting lower parasitemias, while the thin smear is preferred for accurate differentiation of trypanosome species. More sensitive detection is afforded by microscopic examination of the buffy coat following centrifugation.

### *Treatment*

For veterinary use two drugs are commonly administered; Berenil or one of the homidium salts. As resistance to these drugs has been noted, the animals should be observed following treatment. Treatment of human trypanosomiasis is usually by suramin, pentamidine or Berenil, although the prognosis is poor in cases with nervous system involvement. Difluoromethylornithine (eflornithine) is more effective in treating infections that have reached the nervous system.

### *Control*

Control of trypanosomiasis is based upon elimination of the tsetse vector and treatment of affected animals. Presently no vaccine exists or is likely to be developed soon (see section on immune evasion). Vector control is chiefly provided by two means, widespread use of insecticide and destruction of vector habitat. Both of these means have profound environmental consequences.

Due to the tsetse's biology and habits, brush removal and/or deforestation is an effective means of vector control. The tsetse is larviparous, and the young are deposited on the ground underneath vegetation. Removal of brush can therefore deprive the insect of it's habitat and has been quite successful. Unfortunately this is a high maintenance option, to keep the tsetse out, the vegetation must be regularly trimmed. Widespread spraying of insecticides, chiefly DDT and benzene hexachloride, has also been practiced. Although this method can be effective, the benefits must be carefully weighed against known and potential side effects. If must be remembered that neither agent is specific for the tsetse.

Perhaps the most extreme control measure is destruction of reservoir hosts. This was put into practice in East Africa in the 1950's, but was doomed to fail from the outset. Although the larger species of animal hosts could be effectively eliminated, enough small mammals remain to support a tsetse population. When herdsmen brought in cattle the tsetse simply switched to these new hosts. In addition, and not surprisingly, this approach was not popular among conservationists.

### *Trypanotolerance*

Indigenous ruminants in sub-Saharan Africa are also hosts for both *T. brucei* and *T. Congolense,* thus serving as important reservoirs for these parasites. Unlike the severe, usually fatal, course of disease in domestic ruminants, trypanosomes are only mildly pathogenic for the wild ruminants. Likewise, there is a marked difference in the response of different domestic breeds to infection. Some of these, notably the N'Dama cattle (*Bos taurus*) of West Africa, show a considerable degree of innate resistance to infection. This resistance is characterized by a lower parasitemia, and absence of the severe anemia and resultant production loss seen in susceptible hosts. Unfortunately most of the cattle in Africa are not N'Dama, but the trypano-susceptible Zebu type (*Bos indicus*). The humped Zebu cattle have spread over the continent from the east coast, favored by herdsman because of high yields of milk and meat, and this breed's adaptation to semiarid conditions.

Trypanotolerance is an area of increasing scientific interest both for the clues it may provide for new means of prophylaxis and treatment, and for the potential of breeding cattle that combine this resistance with other desirable traits. The exact nature of resistance to trypanosomiasis remains unclear. However recent work has suggested that there are at least two factors at work. In the first place, trypanotolerant animals demonstrate an innate resistance that is evident in the primary attack. In addition it has been suggested that acquired immunity plays an important role under conditions of natural challenge. Supporting the hypothesis of multifactorial resistance is the observation that, crosses between tolerant and susceptible cattle, show an intermediate level of resistance

### *Immune Evasion*

Another area of intense scientific study is this parasite's ability to sequentially present a seemingly endless series of antigens to the immune system. The host's immune system responds vigorously, mounting an attack that eventually eliminates parasites carrying the original antigen. Untouched however, is a population of trypanosomes that have switched antigens, now displaying a different one on their surface. This antigenic variation accounts for the trypanosome's ability to establish chronic infections in the face of a strong immune response. Considerable knowledge about the means by which trypanosomes accomplish this feat has accumulated over the past two decades and is one of the most interesting stories in molecular parasitology. The surface antigen in question is known as the variant-specific surface glycoprotein (VSG) and more than 10 million VSG molecules, all identical, coat the surface of each trypanosome. This coat of VSG molecules is found on the bloodstream forms of the trypanosome and forms a physical barrier protecting the plasma membrane. There are hundreds of separate genes encoding different VSG in the parasite genome, but only one is expressed at a time. There appears to be a loose order of expression of this gene repertoire, with switch rates in natural infections being as high as 1 in 100 cells per division. What this means, in terms of an infected host, is the equivalent of an infection with a new antigenic variant every few days. The VSG proteins and their expression constitute one of the most elegant systems of immune evasion, and a serious challenge for vaccine development.

### *Human Trypanosomiasis*

Trypanosomiasis in humans claims thousands of lives a year, and precludes habitation of highly endemic areas. The causative agents of human trypanosomiasis, *T. brucei gambiense* and *T. brucei rhodesiense*, are morphologically identical to *T. brucei* of cattle. In 1917 however a German researcher named Taute, showed in a rather dramatic fashion, that the agent of nagana was not infective to humans. Taute inoculated native "volunteers" with blood from nagana-afflicted cattle; none of them contracted the dreaded sleeping sickness. In Taute's defense, we must add that he also inoculated himself, though researchers familiar with modern regulations on research involving human subjects still shake their heads in amazement when this story is told.

While *T. brucei* only infects animals, there is solid evidence that *T. brucei rhodesiense* and *T. brucei gambiense* can infect both humans and animals. Animal reservoirs for human trypanosomiasis include primates, wild ungulates and domestic animals. However it is felt that most cases of human trypanosomiasis are the result of human to tsetse to human transmission.

Internet Resources:

The CDC's Department of Parasitic Diseases African Trypanosomiasis Page:
*http://www.cdc.gov/ncidod/dpd/parasites/trypanosomiasis/*

The World Health Organization's The Special Program for Research and Training in Tropical Diseases (TDR) African Trypanosomiasis Page:
*http://www.who.int/tdr/diseases/tryp/default.htm*

American Society for Microbiology News Excerpt on the current status of African Trypanosomiasis:
*http://dev.asmusa.org/International/international-asmnews-Jul00.htm*

CHAPTER 5

# Venezuelan Equine Encephalomyelitis (VEE) and Related Diseases including West Nile Fever in Animals and Humans

*By Dr. Venaye P. Reese*

*Dr. Bob Beede was the author of the original article on Venezuelan Equine Encephalomyelitis. He is a veterinary practitioner in Meridian, Idaho and was formerly Chairman of the Board of Christian Veterinary Mission and is a longtime member of the board*

## VEE—A BRIEF REVIEW AND OVERVIEW

An increasing number of arboviruses (anthropod vector borne viruses) are being recognized worldwide as agents of animal and human disease. Venezuelan Equine Encephalitis (VEE), one of the three most common viruses causing encephalitis in horses in the western hemisphere, has been recognized in two forms in South and Central America for more than 65 years. VEE, Eastern Equine Encephalitis (EEE), and Western Equine Encephalitis (WEE) are all alpha viruses that produce similar central nervous system dysfunction in a variety of vertebrates, including humans and horses commonly called "Sleeping Sickness."

Enzootic forms of VEE are regionally endemic in South, Central and North America and generally cause disease in the mosquito-rodent cycle, and may affect humans, but typically do not cause clinical disease in horses. Epizootic strains, cycling through mosquitos and rodents, also cause serious and sometimes fatal illness in humans and horses of susceptible populations.

A wide-spread outbreak in 1971 spread north through Central America, Mexico and into Texas, USA. Massive vector control programs, large regional quarantines and multiple state equine vaccination programs in the southern states confined the outbreak to parts of Texas. Epizootic VEE has not been diagnosed in the U.S. since 1971.

Substantial outbreaks occurred in southern Mexico in 1993 and 1996. In 1995 following torrential rains and flooding, an outbreak occurred in Venezuela and Northern Columbia. It involved 13,000 human cases and an undetermined number of deaths.

An outbreak in Columbia, South America in the summer of 1998, originally thought to be VEE, based on IgM antibody titers in equine, upon virus identification was actually found to be strains of EEE enzootic virus. Several minor outbreaks (most identified as slightly mutated enzootic strains of VEE) have occurred in Mexico and the Columbia/Venezuela areas in recent years but have been contained. Since 1993, VEE activity has resulted in increased security measures at the Mexico/U.S. border during periods of outbreak.

### *VEE—Etiology and Epidemiology*

The natural reservoir for VEE virus is thought to be wild birds and rodents and other small vertebrates. The disease is transmitted by mosquitos and other blood sucking insects. Unlike EEE and WEE, horses may serve as an important amplifier of epidemic VEE, producing a viremia (blood level of virus) sufficient to infect mosquitos through allowing transmission of the disease by blood transfer. In addition, horses may spread the disease to other horses by contact or aerosol since the virus is concentrated in the salivary glands. It is questionable as to whether horse to human transmission occurs in this way.

VEE is concentrated in areas having the combination of reservoir hosts and mosquitos. It occurs more commonly in pastured than stabled horses. Recent outbreaks occurred in areas of flooding which contained a susceptible population of horses, burros and mules lacking current VEE vaccination. Enzootic subtypes of VEE are less likely to spread and generally do not affect horses. Epizootic subtypes may spread rapidly and are highly pathogenic to horses.

### *VEE Symptoms*

In horses, clinical signs occur approximately 5 days after infection and may include fever, impaired vision, irregular gait, wandering, reduced reflexes, circling, hanging lower lip, inability to swallow and head pressing. Symptoms may progress, with increasing paralysis, inability to rise, convulsions and death occurring in two to three days. Mildly affected animals may slowly recover in a few weeks, but may be left with residual brain damage. Mortality (death) in horses with VEE can reach 50% to 75%.

Differential diagnoses are very important and continue to increase in number. Other viral threats to human and horse health include Rabies, EEE, WEE, or one of the lesser known viruses such as Highlands J (HG) (variation of WEE). The spread to the western hemisphere of *West Nile Virus to the U.S. (New York in 1999, 12 Eastern states and Canada, by end of 2000) and the emergence in other parts of the world of encephalitis viruses (Morbilli virus—Australia) and the frightening outbreak of what is now named Nipah virus in Malaysia in 1998 (originally thought to be Japanese Encephalitis) reinforce the importance of alert surveillance and rapid and correct diagnosis and containment of this type of disease.

Additionally, non-viral etiologics such as hepatoencephalopathy (liver-brain disorder), bacterial encephalitis and such etiologies as tetanus and botulism must be considered. Equine protozoal mycloencephalitis (EPM) a protozoal brain disorder, verminous encephalitis (parasite migration), leukoencephalomalacia (fumonesin toxicity from ingesting moldy corn) must be considered. Except for morbilli, Nipah, JE, and African Horse Sickness (eastern hemisphere) and West Nile (currently limited to Eastern U.S.), these conditions exist in areas where VEE is known to occur.

Differential diagnosis is frequently made initially by testing blood for antibodies to the virus, followed by virus isolations and identification by laboratory. New PCR techniques are improving ID methods.

### *VEE Treatment*

No specific antiviral drugs are available. Supportive treatment including anti-inflammatory drugs (phenylbutazone, lamime), seizure control with sedatives (don't forget that some tranquilizers, such as acepromazine, may actually preapilate or exaggerate seizuring), and intensive nursing care may help mild cases. A slow IV administration of 99% DMSO mixed in a 10% solution of saline at the rate of 1 cc per kg, may be repeated daily for 2–3 days and may help stabilize central nervous system tissue damage by reducing brain edema. Prevention of body sores and insect attacks is important for recumbent animals in humid climates.

### *VEE Prevention and Control*

During outbreaks, the most effective way to prevent further spread of the disease is to quarantine infected and exposed equines and initiate vaccination of susceptible equids and carry out mosquito control measures. Prevention is the best and most cost effective method of control for any disease problem. Since VEE is mainly spread by mosquitos, mosquito control measures are very helpful, (i.e., drainage of standing water, treatment of mosquito breeding areas and insect repellant use on horses).

Stabling horses and spraying or screening against mosquitos is advisable during outbreaks. In many instances, mosquito control may be next to impossible. Vaccines are therefore the most effective single method of prevention and control in the face of an outbreak. Horses, mules and burros in high risk areas should be vaccinated one month prior to mosquito season. They may require a booster every six months in regions with extended mosquito seasons.

Although research shows evidence of possible cross protection for VEE in EEE and WEE vaccinated horses, VEE vaccine is recommended for horses with high risk of exposure to VEE. In 1996, the American Association of Equine Practitioners (AAEP) in U.S. recommended U.S. horses in states bordering Mexico receive VEE vaccinations, with some qualification concerning export restrictions on horses with VEE titers. Veterinarians are advised to consider vaccination carefully and keep complete and accurate records of vaccinated animals to minimize confusion.

A new vaccine (TC-83) for humans is currently being tested and given to individuals who are at risk of repeated exposure in the lab and field.

Suspicious encephalitis cases in equine and humans should be reported immediately to Government Animal Health-Regulatory Officials. Detection of an outbreak is critical for effective containment and to limit economic loss. Quarantine of infected and exposed animals in an area where VEE is occurring is often necessary for control of an outbreak. International movement of horses is frequently restricted while epidemics are controlled and active disease eliminated.

Animal Health personnel in North, Central and South America have increased surveillance and rapid cooperative response to VEE and EEE in recent years. Health officials are concerned with both the possibilities of enzootic shift to epizootic strains of VEE and EEE and the recognized threat of newly emerging viruses of zoonotic potential. Rapid action by owners and practicing veterinarians is critical as the first line of defense to alert officials of encephalitis cases early in outbreaks.

### *VEE in Humans*

Clinical manifestations of this viral infection are influenza-like, with an abrupt onset of severe headache, chills, fever, myalgia, retro-orbital pain, nausea and vomiting. Conjunctival and pharyngeal injections are the only physical signs. Most infections are relatively mild, with symptoms lasting 3–5 days. Some cases may have a diphasic fever course; after a few days of fever, particularly in children, CNS involvement may appear, ranging from somnolence to frank encephalitis with disorientation, paralysis, coma and death. During the 1971 Texas, USA outbreak, 3 of 40 patients studied had severe CNS involvement, with sequelae of personality change and/or paralysis.

Diagnosis is suspected on clinical and epidemiologic grounds (exposure in an area of an equine epizootic antibody titer or specific IgM). Virus can be isolated in cell culture from blood and nasopharyngeal washings during the first 72 hours of symptoms; acute and convalescent sera 10 days apart reveal a rising antibody titer. Laboratory infections may occur unless proper containment facilities are used.

There is no specific treatment.

### *West Nile Virus*

*West Nile Virus, never found in the western hemisphere before 1999, is a flavivirus most commonly found in Africa, western Asia, the Middle East and Mediterranean Europe. The virus is transmitted by mosquitos that acquire it from infected birds. A number of other species may harbor subclinical infections when bitten by a virus-laden mosquito, but humans and horses may suffer clinical illness with significant morbidity and mortality. Both humans and horses are considered most likely dead end hosts not capable of producing high viremia for transmission by mosquito bite. Contact or aerosol transfer of this disease is not thought probable from horses or humans, but there is some evidence contact transmission is possible between infected and noninfected birds (crows). A vaccine is being developed.

The discovery of this virus (which closely resembles St. Louis Encephalitis Virus, endemic in the U.S. and affecting birds and humans) in New York in the fall of 1999, resulted in massive surveillance and control efforts on the entire eastern seaboard of the United States. It is believed the virus was accidently introduced by birds or mosquitos brought in carrying the virus. Efforts to eliminate the virus have been unsuccessful, and since the virus survived overwintering in the winter of 1999–2000, and re-emerged in the summer of 2000, it is generally accepted that the U.S. will be dealing with an ongoing disease problem with West Nile Virus.

**Information obtained from: Same as original article, plus recent personal communication with Dr. Tim Cordes, USDA-APHIS-VS Equine Disease Staff; USDA 1998 Summary of Equine Encephalitis Surveillance; Cross-protective immunity between equine encephalomyelitis viruses in equids, Walter TE, Jochim MM, Barber TL, Thompson, LH, Am J Vet Res 1989 Sep; 50(9); Medically important arboviruses of the United States and Canada, Calisher CH, Clin Microbiol Rev 1994 Jan; 7(1); Emergence of a new epidemic/epizootic Venezuelan equine encephalitis virus in South America, Rico-Hesse R, Weaver SC, deSiger J, Medina G, Salas RA, Proc Natl Acad Sci USA 1995 June 6; 92(12); Antibodies to arthropod-borne encephalitis viruses in small mammals from southern Florida, Day JF, Stark LM, Zhang JT, Ramsey AM, Scott TW, J Wildl Dis 1996 Jul; 32(3); Update: West Nile Virus Activity-Eastern United States, 2000, MMWR Nov 20, 2000, Vol. 49/No. 46, pp 1044–1047; Epi Notes Disease Prevention and Epidemiology Newsletter, Vol. XXI No. 1, March-April 2000, SC Department of Health and Environmental Control.*

CHAPTER 6

# Rift Valley Fever in Animals and Humans

*By Dr. John C. Morrill*

## RIFT VALLEY FEVER: A ZOONOTIC DISEASE HISTORY AND REVIEW

Rift Valley fever virus (Family Bunyaviridae, genus Phlebovirus) is unique among the phleboviruses in its pathogenicity for humans and domestic animals, its various routes of infection, and its wide host range. Since the first isolation of the virus and a detailed description of the disease in sheep in the Rift Valley of Kenya in 1930, there have been significant epizootics in South Africa, Egypt in 1977 and 1993, West Africa in 1987, Madagascar in 1990, Kenya and Somalia in 1997–1998, and most recently in Mauritania in 1998. Presently, virologic and serologic evidence suggests that the virus exists throughout sub-Saharan Africa and Madagascar and, in light of its recurrence in Egypt in 1993, may be extending its range even further. In September 2000, cases of unexplained hemorrhagic fever in humans and associated animal deaths in southwestern Saudi Arabia and Yemen were confirmed as Rift Valley Fever. Mid January 2001, Rift Valley Fever had claimed 227 lives in Saudi Arabia and Yemen. This outbreak on the Arabian Peninsula represents the first cases of RVF outside Africa.

The virus is typically associated with pastoral regions where habitat conducive to the maintenance of arthropod vectors is present. Natural hosts for RVF virus include mosquitoes, ruminants, and humans. Newborn lambs, calves, and puppies are highly susceptible.

### *Rift Valley Fever in Humans*

The disease in humans is usually a temporarily incapacitating illness. Infection results in fever, malaise, headache, and myalgia, often with other constitutional symptoms developing, followed by complete recovery. Probably 1% or less of human infections progress to encephalitis, retinal disease, or the more severe and often fatal complications of hemorrhagic disease. The determinants of these different syndromes are unknown. During the RVF virus outbreak in Egypt in 1993, a presumptive case definition of ocular disease characterized by macular and paramacular retinal lesions, frequently with hemorrhage and edema, following a febrile episode was established. This clinical presentation was quite different from the previous outbreak in 1977–1978 in which the hemorrhagic form was frequently seen and accounted for nearly 600 human deaths.

Complications of encephalitis and retinal disease usually develop as the acute illness fades, or during the recovery period. The hemorrhagic fever syndrome seen in an estimated 1% of human cases has a case fatality of approximately 50% and is manifested during the course of acute illness. Patients with hemorrhagic disease develop petechial, mucous membrane and gastrointestinal bleeding. They become jaundiced and die in shock. Disseminated vascular damage and hepatic failure probably contribute to the patient's demise.

The introduction of RVF virus in Egypt in 1977 produced the largest recorded RVF epidemic. Before this epidemic only four human deaths attributable to RVF had been reported. The sudden and unexpected appearance of this previously geographically limited sub-Saharan virus and the unprecedented numbers of encephalitic, ocular, and fatal hemorrhagic disease remains an enigma. Introduction by means of importation of diseased animals from the south or wind-borne arthropods are unproven possibilities. Although extensive epidemiological data could not be collected, an estimated 18,000 to >200,000 clinical cases in humans occurred with 598 fatalities and about 800 cases of ocular disease associated with RVF virus infection. Animal losses due to abortion and mortality were high and impacted significantly on the availability and cost of animal protein in Egypt.

### *Epidemiology of Rift Valley Fever*

Epidemics of RVF typically center around regions where there are large concentrations of sheep and cattle. Explosive epidemics occur periodically and are usually associated with periods of heavy rainfall producing localized flooding and dense or expanding vector populations. Transovarially infected floodwater *Aedes* eggs hatch, producing infected adults that feed extensively on cattle. Other mosquito species feeding on infected livestock ingest viremic blood meals and, if those mosquitoes are efficient vectors, become competent secondary vectors. *Culicoides spp.* and sand flies may play limited roles in biological and mechanical transmission.

In the absence of epidemics, a cycle of enzootic circulation exists in many regions of Africa. Livestock infections, probably acquired by the bite of infected mosquitoes, result in low rates of disease and abortion that are undiagnosed due to confusion with other livestock diseases as well as a lack of diagnostic capabilities. Reservoirs for RVF virus are unidentified, though there is strong evidence of interepidemic maintenance via transovarial transmission in certain *Aedes* mosquitoes. The infected eggs are deposited and may remain dormant in depressions, called "dambos" in East Africa, that are subject to inundation. When flooding occurs, the eggs hatch and infected larvae emerge and develop into infected adults.

Although aerosol transmission between infected and susceptible livestock appears less important than mosquito transmission, humans may be infected by aerosol in the laboratory and during slaughter of viremic animals. Blood, serum, and the products of abortion from RVF virus-infected animals are sources for infection of humans in at-risk occupations such as abattoir workers, farmers, veterinarians, and laboratory technicians. The major natural means of RVF virus transmission is by bite of infected mosquitoes, but mechanical transmission by arthropods is possible. Consumption of milk or meat from infected animals does not appear to be a common means of transmission.

Clinical signs vary considerably and disease progression and severity of disease are generally inversely proportional to age. Adult cattle and sheep may suffer mortality rates of 10–30% or higher, depending on the nutritional state of the animal; but in animals fewer than 7 days old, fatality rates may approach 100%. The disease is characterized by a short incubation period, fever, hepatitis, abortion, and death. Widespread abortion, infertility and rapidly fatal neonatal disease are typical of outbreaks among cattle and sheep. Other overt signs are inconsistent, but include congestion of mucous membranes, injected conjunctiva, hyperemia of the oral mucosa, mucopurulent nasal discharge, salivation, vomiting, anorexia, general weakness, an unsteady gait, fetid diarrhea, and a rapid decrease in milk production. A definite leukopenia, most severe in younger animals, which corresponds to maximal viremia and temperature response, is seen, often followed by leukocytosis in later stages of the disease. Elevated serum AST, GGT and LDH values are common.

Experimentally infected animals are viremic for 2 to 5 days with titers often in excess of $10^8$ plaque-forming units per ml (PFU/ml). No long-term carrier state in animals has been identified. Central nervous system involvement, evidenced by encephalitis, occurs periodically in experimentally infected rodents.

While the incidence of encephalitis in cattle naturally infected with RVF virus is not known, there is a single report of RVF viral encephalomyelitis in an experimentally infected calf.

The most consistent pathologic changes in all species affected involve the liver. The liver appears to be the primary site of virus replication, and initial mild hepatocellular changes rapidly progress to final massive necrosis. Hepatic lesions in adult ruminants are not as severe as those found in neonates, but multiple necrotic areas may be present. Coagulated blood may be found in the lumen of the gallbladder in those cases with marked hemorrhage in the liver. Hemorrhages are seen infrequently in abomasum and intestinal tract.

### *Diagnosis of Rift Valley Fever*

An epidemiological pattern suggestive of RVF includes short incubation period; high mortality in lambs, calves, and kids that are less than 1 week old; illness in adult sheep and cattle; high abortion rates among cows and ewes; liver lesions at necropsy; acute febrile disease in humans; and the presence of dense populations of arthropod vectors.

In the laboratory, a characteristic histopathological finding of liver necrosis in all susceptible animals often provides the first clue that the disease is RVF. A definitive diagnosis of RVF is accomplished by isolating and identifying the virus or by observing a fourfold rise in specific, neutralizing antibody titer between acute and convalescent sera. During past epizootics, the most common material used for virus isolation included whole blood or serum collected from animals at the peak of pyrexia. Fresh specimens of liver from animals dying of the illness and the products of abortion are also excellent diagnostic materials. Infected humans are also a source of diagnostic material, and, if possible, suspected mosquito vectors should be collected for virus-isolation studies.

RVF virus may be isolated in laboratory rodents as well as in a number of common cell culture systems; however, virus isolation should not be attempted unless adequate personal protection, such as vaccination, can be assured or biosafety level 3 (BSL-3) containment facilities are available.

Serological techniques used to demonstrate RVF virus antibody in domestic animals and humans include HI, CF, IFA, agar gel diffusion, plaque-reduction neutralization, and ELISA tests. The ELISA is also used to demonstrate viral antigen in suspect tissue and serum. The utility of polymerase chain reaction (PCR) methodology as a diagnostic tool for RVF virus is being evaluated.

### *Treatment and Control of Rift Valley Fever*

No specific treatments are currently available. The presence of serum antibody to RVF virus seems to be the major immunological defense mechanism in recovery. In rodents and monkeys, the outcome of RVF virus infection appears to be regulated by serum antibody, and interferon may be a contributory factor in limiting viremia and preventing clinical disease. Passive antibody therapy, by administration of immune plasma or serum, may be effective but impractical in an epizootic. Neonatal calves have been shown to be completely protected against experimental challenge with virulent virus through ingestion of colostrum from immune dams.

Relocating animals to an altitude where mosquitoes are absent or applying residual insecticides to animals and their pens and barns has been suggested, though movement of animals during an epizootic is undesirable and rarely practical, and effectiveness of residual insecticides in animal-holding areas depends on vector habits. Limiting amplification of virus in domestic animals will probably block extensive human disease, and mass vaccination is the method of choice in controlling RVF during an epizootic.

Effective live-attenuated and killed veterinary vaccines for RVF are used in many African countries. The live-attenuated

Smithburn strain provides long-lasting immunity but is abortogenic in pregnant ewes. The live-virus vaccines should be used only in enzootic areas of Africa or to control an epizootic.

Killed vaccines are recommended for outside enzootic areas of Africa. A formalin-inactivated vaccine is safe for pregnant ewes but provides only short-term immunity and requires booster inoculations to maintain a durable immunity. Stringent production controls are necessary to ensure the absence of residual live virus.

The only vaccine cleared for human use is a killed product available only from the United States Army Medical Research and Material Command (USAMRMC). This vaccine is in limited supply and requires an initial three-dose series for protective immunity with annual booster inoculations required to maintain that immunity.

A live, attenuated vaccine (MP-12) developed for use in humans and livestock is being tested. Extensive laboratory studies have shown this vaccine to be safe and efficacious against virulent virus challenge in pregnant cows and ewes as well as in neonatal calves and lambs. Presently, the current lot of MP-12 vaccine is undergoing human testing at the United States Army Medical Research Institute of Infectious Diseases (USAMRIID).

Suggested specific measures to control a Rift Valley Fever epidemic include:

1. Implement an animal vaccination program.
   a. Establish a vaccine barrier between known affected areas and unaffected areas.
   b. Positively identify vaccinated animals with a means of identification not easily counterfeited or duplicated.
   c. Prohibit the use of common needles for immunization.
   d. Prohibit the movement of non-vaccinated animals from affected areas.
   e. Employ integrated vector control measures. Use caution to prevent destruction of mosquito predator species as well as contamination of water and food supplies.
   f. Use personal protective measures such as insect sprays, repellents, and bed nets.

2. Implement active disease surveillance as well as seroprevalence outside the area of active virus transmission.
   a. Inform human health care providers and veterinarians of the present epizootic/epidemic and be alert for cases exhibiting common signs and sequelae of the disease.
   b. Alert those in high-risk occupations to the potential hazard of infection through activities such as patient contact, the slaughtering of sick animals, and assisting with abortions in ruminants.
   c. Increase public awareness of the threat.
3. Vaccination of persons in high risk occupations.

CHAPTER 7

# Anthrax in Animals and Humans

*By Dr. Keith Flanagan*

## ANTHRAX

(Wool sorters disease, Malignant edema, Malignant pustules, Charbon, Splenic fever)

Anthrax is an acute infectious disease of great economic and public health importance. It is most common in food animals, but can affect a wide range of warm-blooded animals, including man. It is found *worldwide* and is caused by the spore forming bacteria *Bacillus anthracis.* It is most prevalent in developing countries where control programs have not been established. Outbreaks occur most often in low-lying areas where the soil pH is greater than 6 (alkaline soils). Secondary outbreaks can also be traced to contaminated animal products such as animal-origin feeds and fertilizer, hides, milk, meat, and wool.

### *Pathogen*

The etiologic agent of anthrax is *Bacillus anthracis,* a member of the genus Bacillus. *B. anthracis* is an aeorbic, large (1–1.2 by 3–5 microns), capsulated Gram positive rod that grows in chains. It is non-motile, non-hemolytic and produces spores that are resistant to heat, ultraviolet light and many disinfectants. The organism is susceptible to penicillin and its derivatives. The robust spore enables the disease to persist.

There is a lack of molecular polymorphism within *B. anthracis*. Analysis using amplified fragment length polymorphisms (AFIP) observed only some 30 differences among >1000 fragments. A comparative DNA sequencing study of the protective antigen gene found only five differences across 2500 nucleotides in 25 diverse strains. An exception to this trend was the work of Andersen and colleagues who examined a previously identified PCR marker by DNA sequence analysis. They found that a large open reading frame (*vrrA*) contained a variable number tandemly repeated (VNTR) sequence. Five different allelic states have been observed in the *vrrA* VNTR among diverse strains. To date VNTR's appear to contain greater diversity and hence, greater discrimination capacity than any other type of molecular typing system. Using eight different VNTR markers—six in the chromosome and one in each plasmid—it is possible to distinguish some 89 unique strains world wide. As further variable regions are identified, new VNTR markers will add increasing clarity to the genetic diversity of *B. anthracis*.

Using this system it has been possible to demonstrate a worldwide series of strains, Group A, and a more limited series, Group B, to date found largely only in southern Africa. These are genetically and epidemiologically different. Speculatively Group B may be the original pathogen—with the domestication of ruminant livestock and their entry into Africa, it adapted to these new hosts and nomadic husbandry, becoming Group A; then was exported to the Middle East and Asian countries.

### *Toxins*

The pathogenicity of *B. anthracis* is due to two plasmids, pX01 and pX02; pX01 encodes a tripartite toxin and pX02 is responsible for the poly-D-glutamic acid capsule which protects the bacteria from phagocytosis. The toxin complex consists of three interacting thermolabile proteins produced during the log phase of growth. These are known as protective antigen (PA, 83kDa), edema factor (EF, 87kDa), and lethal factor (LF, 89kDa).

PA induces protective antitoxic antibodies and is the central binding element for anthrax toxin. EF is necessary for the edema producing activity of the toxin and is an adenylate cyclase. LF is essential for the lethal effects of the anthrax toxin. On their own these three factors exhibit no significant biological activity other than antigenicity.

The anthrax toxin and capsule are thought to play a role in the early stages of infection through their direst effects on phagocytes. The spores are phagocytized by macrophages where germination and multiplication occurs. The vegetative bacilli kill the macrophage, and release live as extracellular pathogens, and reach high numbers in the bloodstream (up to $10^8$ bacilli per mL have been recorded).

Expression of the anthrax toxin, during the growth and expansion of the disease within the host's body, is regulated by body temperature and $CO_2$ concentrations. The toxin proteins are then secreted into the host's bloodstream and carried through the body. Most cell types have surface receptors for PA; for example a mouse macrophage may have as many as 30,000 receptors per cell. PA binds to these receptors and is activated by a host protease which cleaves off a 20kDa piece exposing a secondary receptor site for which EF and LF compete to bind. The PA + LF and/or PA+EF are then internalized into the cell by receptor-mediated endocytosis and EF and LF are released into the cytosol of the host's cell. This induces the cell to release cytokines and to undergo an oxidative burst before dying.

### *The Disease*

Most commonly, outbreaks occur in grazing animals during the warm season when minimal temperatures are above 16° C following marked climatic or ecological changes such as flooding or drought. The flooding is thought to concentrate the spores in low-lying areas and then, during the drought, the animals graze closer to the ground. There is usually a history of previous outbreaks in the area, although several years may elapse between outbreaks. The spores of anthrax are extremely resistant to temperature, sunlight, drying, and chemical disinfectants. They can live for years in the soil until climatic conditions (humidity, pH, and temperature) are ideal for its transformation to the more infective vegetative form. Grazing animals are more likely to be infected. Flies and other biting insects may also mechanically transmit anthrax from one animal to another during an outbreak, but this is probably of minor importance.

### *Clinical Disease in Animals*

Clinical signs generally appear 3 to 7 days after ingestion of the bacteria, and the course of the disease varies from peracute, to acute, to chronic. In cattle, sheep, and goats the course may be peracute and an animal that appeared normal only a few hours earlier may be found dead. In the acute form there is a very rapid onset of fever (up to 42° C). The animal may stagger, tremble and have signs of abdominal pain and respiratory distress. One often sees blood-tinged diarrhea and blood in the urine and milk, as well as hemorrhage from the mouth and nose. Pregnant animals may abort. Death may occur within 24 hours with convulsions in the terminal stages. The acute form is more common in cattle, sheep, and horses.

In swine, the disease tends to be more chronic with swelling in the head and neck region. This can often interfere with breathing and swallowing and the animal may die from asphyxia. There may be blood-tinged mucous discharge from the mouth and nose. The chronic form may also be seen in horses and dogs. These cases are more responsive to antibiotic treatment.

Lesions: (NOTE: If anthrax is suspected, *do not perform a postmortem exam!*)

Rigor mortis is usually absent or incomplete with dark blood oozing from the mouth, nose and anus. There is marked bloating and rapid decomposition. Even though one should not open the carcass, the owners often try to salvage what they can of the animal. The blood will be dark and it fails to clot. Hemorrhages may be seen through the abdomen and thorax and on the surface of most of the organs, especially the heart and intestines. The spleen usually is enlarged and resembles blackberry jam. Hemorrhages and edema of the pharyngeal area and tonsils is present in the chronic forms.

### *Diagnosis*

Anthrax can resemble other conditions that cause sudden death. In cattle and sheep this includes clostridial infections, bloat, and lightning strike. Also acute leptospirosis, bacillary hemoglobinuria, anaplasmosis, babesiosis and acute poisonings by bracken fern, sweet clover, lead and blue-green algae must be considered in cattle. In horses, acute infectious anemia, colic, lightning, lead poisoning and blue-green algae toxicity may resemble anthrax. In swine, hog cholera, African swine fever, and pharyngeal malignant edema must also be considered.

Diagnosis is usually based on clinical signs as well as a past history of anthrax in the area, but this may be difficult in a new area. Laboratory confirmation may be necessary. A small amount of blood collected by syringe from the jugular or other superficial vessel is best. Before shipping, the lab should be notified to determine the best method of shipping and to ascertain whether it is equipped to handle anthrax.

Blood and edema fluid smears stained with polychrome methylene blue should reveal short chains of large gram positive rods. They will have a characteristic pink capsule around the blue-black square ended bacilli. Bacteriological cultures or animal inoculations may not be reliable if antibiotics were given to the sick animal. Many labs may be equipped with proper ventilation to prevent accidental laboratory exposure to humans. There is a fluorescent antibody test to detect capsular production, but it may not be available in many developing countries. Western blot and ELISA test for antibody detection may be of little value in acute cases.

### *Treatment*

Anthrax is highly susceptible to several antibiotics. Penicillin and oxytetracycline are very effective and easily available in most countries. The recommended daily dose of penicillin for swine, goats, and sheep is 22,000 units/kg and the daily dose for cattle is 5 to 10 million units. Therapy should be continued for at least 5 days and the daily dose should be administered in 2 equal parts at 12-hour intervals for at least the first two days. If potassium penicillin or sodium penicillin is available, it should be given IV as the initial dose in severely ill animals.

The daily oxytetracycline dose is 4.5 mg/kg for all species and should be divided into two equal parts every 12 hours for the first two days. It may be given IM or IV (slowly) for at least 5 days. Other antibiotics that may be effective are amoxicillin, doxycycline, erythromycin, and gentamicin. Antibiotics should not be given to healthy animals for at least seven days after vaccination against anthrax since the vaccine is a modified live vaccine.

Hyper-immune anthrax serum is recommended for use along with antibiotic therapy, but may not be locally available.

### *Clinical Signs in Humans*

There are three recognized forms of anthrax in humans: cutaneous, pulmonary, and gastrointestinal. Rare cases of anthrax meningitis have also been documented in Haiti.

The cutaneous form is the most common form and accounts for over 90% of the cases in humans. It has an incubation period of 2 to 5 days after inoculation of a spore or vegetative bacilli into a wound. A reddened papular lesion develops and is commonly mistaken for an insect bite. This develops into a blister and later into a characteristic painless black and depressed ulcer. Edema in the area is marked and the edema often extends to the associated lymph nodes and beyond. A lesion on the head or neck can often result in laryngeal swelling so severe that a tracheal tube must be placed to insure a clear air passage. Mortality is low if treated quickly, but can approach 20% in untreated cases.

The pulmonary form has an incubation period of 1 to 5 days after inhaling the anthrax spores. It begins like many common respiratory infections with a fever, malaise, muscle pain and a cough. In the second phase 3 to 5 days later, the patient suddenly develops respiratory distress, sweating, cyanosis, shock and death within 24 hours. Mortality is close to 100%.

The incubation period of the gastrointestinal form is 12 hours to 5 days after eating contaminated meat. The patient develops fever, vomiting, bloody diarrhea, and malaise. Mortality can be close to 50%.

The treatment of choice in humans is usually penicillin. Tetracyclines and erythromycin are effective if used early and are the drug of choice for patients with penicillin allergy. A recent intelligence report indicates that a genetically engineered strain of anthrax that is resistant to penicillin and doxycycline has been developed for biological warfare in Russia. However, it is sensitive to ciprofloxacin.

A cell free vaccine is available and is recommended for high risk persons such as veterinarians or those handling potentially contaminated raw materials such as meats, hides, or wool.

### *Prevention and Control*

The best method of prevention is to prevent the release of additional organisms into the environment. The carcass, bedding, and other contaminated materials and soil should be quickly burned or deeply buried on a site when possible. It is best to burn the carcass in a pit. Old tires may be of benefit to add additional heat for the burning process. If buried, the carcass and surrounding areas should be covered with quicklime (calcium oxide). The carcass should not be opened. The vegetative form of the bacteria is usually destroyed inside the decomposing carcass. Once opened and exposed to air, the vegetative form transforms to the resistant spores and a new area of infectivity is now seeded. Predators should be kept away from the carcass until burning or burying. They can play a role in the spread of the spores into new areas.

Vaccination is the preferred method for preventing future cases of anthrax in an affected area. Vaccine should be given at least 2 to 4 weeks before the normal seasonal outbreaks. The Sterne vaccine is accepted as the standard for anthrax vaccines. It is an avirulent, non-encapsulated B. Anthracis vaccine that induces immunity within 7 days. A booster in 2 to 4 weeks may be beneficial in highly endemic areas, but field studies have shown that an annual booster is adequate. Owners should be warned that localized subcutaneous edema near the injection site may develop within 24 hours and may last several days. Animals should not be given antibiotics for seven days after vaccination or the effect of the vaccine may be negated. Food animals should not be vaccinated within 60 days of slaughter and milk from unvaccinated febrile animals in the area should be properly destroyed. Sick animals in the affected area should be isolated, and healthy animals moved to a new area and quarantined for two weeks.

The herd should be checked three times a day for sick animals—rapid breathing, fever or other relevant signs—for one or two weeks. These should be separated and treated with antibiotics. Animals do respond well to treatment even when far advanced.

*All cases should be reported to the proper Agriculture and Public Health officials.*

### *Addendum: Update on Anthrax Treatment*

The following information is the most up to date material on the treatment of Anthrax. Since it represents an advance in treatment we thought it would be well to include it.

It was developed from information gathered from treatment of cases following terrorist activity in the USA in 2001.

| *Category* | *Initial Therapy (intravenous)*[§,¶] | *Duration* |
|---|---|---|
| Adults | Ciprofloxacin 400 mg every 12 hrs*<br>**or**<br>Doxycycline 100 mg every 12 hrs[††]<br>**and**<br>One or two additional antimicrobials[¶] | IV treatment initially**. Switch to oral antimicrobial therapy when clinically appropriate:<br>Ciprofloxacin 500mg po BID<br>**or**<br>Doxycycline 100 mg po BID<br>Continue for 60 days (IV and po combined)[§§] |
| Children | Ciprofloxacin 10–15 mg/kg every 12 hrs[¶¶,***]<br>**or**<br>Doxycycline:[†††,††]<br>>8 yrs and >45 kg: 100 mg every 12 hrs<br>>8 yrs and ≤45 kg: 2.2 mg/kg every 12 hrs<br>≤8 yrs: 2.2 mg/kg every 12 hrs<br>**and**<br>One or two additional antimicrobials[¶] | IV treatment initially**. Switch to oral antimicrobial therapy when clinically appropriate:<br>Ciprofloxacin 10–15 mg/kg po every 12 hrs***<br>**or**<br>Doxycycline:[†††]<br>>8 yrs and >45 kg: 100 mg po BID<br>>8 yrs and ≤45 kg: 2.2 mg/kg po BID<br>≤8 yrs: 2.2 mg/kg po BID<br>Continue for 60 days (IV and po combined)[§§] |
| Pregnant women [§§§] | Same for nonpregnant adults (the high death rate from the infection outweighs the risk posed by the antimicrobial agent) | IV treatment initially. Switch to oral antimicrobial therapy when clinically appropriate.[†] Oral therapy regimens same for nonpregnant adults |

| *Category* | *Initial Therapy (intravenous)§¶* | *Duration* |
|---|---|---|
| Immunocompromised persons | Same for nonimmunocompromised persons and children | Same for nonimmunocompromised persons and children |

*For gastrointestinal and Oropharyngeal Anthrax, use regimens recommended for Inhalational Anthrax.

†Ciprofloxacin or Doxycycline should be considered an essential part of first-line therapy for inhalational anthrax.

§Steroids may be considered as an adjunct therapy for patients with severe edema and for meningitis based on experience with bacterial meningitis of other etiologies.

¶Other agents with *in vitro* activity include Rifampin, Vancomycin, Penicillin, Ampicillin, Chloramphenicol, Imipenem, Clindamycin, and Clarithromycin. Because of concerns of constitutive and inducible beta-lactamases in *Bacillus anthracis,* Penicillin and Ampicillin should not be used alone. Consultation with an infectious disease specialist is advised.

**Initial therapy may be altered based on clinical course of the patient; one or two antimicrobial agents (e.g., Ciprofloxacin or Doxycycline) may be adequate as the patient improves.

††If meningitis is suspected, Doxycycline may be less optimal because of poor central nervous system penetration.

§§Because of the potential persistence of spores after an aerosol exposure, antimicrobial therapy should be continued for 60 days.

¶¶If intravenous Ciprofloxacin is not available, oral ciprofloxacin may be acceptable because it is rapidly and well absorbed from the gastrointestinal tract with no substantial loss by first-pass metabolism. Maximum serum concentrations are attained 1–2 hours after oral dosing but may not be achieved if vomiting or ileus are present.

***In children, Ciprofloxacin dosage should not exceed 1 g/day.

†††The American Academy of Pediatrics recommends treatment of young children with Tetracyclines for serious infections (e.g. Rocky Mountain Spotted Fever).

§§§Although Tetracyclines are not recommended during pregnancy, their use may be indicated for life-threatening illness. Adverse effects on developing teeth and bones are dose related; therefore, Doxycycline might be used for a short time (7–14 days) before 6 months of gestation.

From Communicable Disease Center, Atlanta, GA, USA Morbidity and Mortality Weekly Report. October 26, 2001/Vol.50/No. 42

CHAPTER 8

# Leptospirosis in Animals and Humans

*By Dr. John R. Cole*

## LEPTOSPIROSIS—HISTORY AND REVIEW

Leptospirosis was first described in Germany in the 1880's by Weil who had observed a febrile illness and jaundice in a patient. Reports of cases continued in Europe throughout the latter part of the 1800's, most describing jaundice, fever, enlargement of the liver and spleen, and renal involvement. The etiology of "Weil's Disease" was unknown until 1914 when Japanese investigators observed spirochetes in the liver of guinea pigs that had been injected with blood from patients with symptoms of this disease. These Japanese investigators named the organism *Spirochaeta icterohemorrhagiae.* Within two years, German researchers observed spirochetes in organ specimens and British scientists confirmed the transmission experiment in guinea pigs described earlier by the Japanese. These are very slender, helical organisms have a characteristic hook in one or both ends.

In 1907 the first reported cased of Leptospirosis in the United States occurred in Louisiana. The patient at the time was diagnosed clinically to have yellow fever, but thirty years later the illness was confirmed as leptospirosis.

As awareness of the disease increased, additional leptrospiral serotypes were isolated worldwide from humans and animals during the 1920's and 1930's. At least 50 serotypes were named by the 1950's, and more than 250 by the late 1990's.

Historically, the disease has been observed in sewer workers and people swimming in water contaminated with infected urine, or workers in cane fields, abattoirs, or milking parlors. In domesticated animals the disease is generally transmitted by direct or indirect exposure to infected urine, usually contaminated water.

### *Leptospirosis in Humans*

Leptospirosis is a zoonotic disease that has been reported in humans *throughout the world.* It is transmitted to man through the skin or mucous membranes, after direct or indirect contact with urine from infected animals. Chief reservoirs for the leptospires are rats, other wild rodents, dogs, cattle, and swine.

The infection in man is generally an acute septicemic disease with symptoms ranging from a mild flu-like illness to a more severe condition that includes jaundice, renal insufficiency, meningitis, and death. It is usually characterized by two phases: first, a leptospiremia for about seven days with chills, headaches, high fever and myalgia; and second, an "immune" phase lasting several weeks. In the immune phase, there is a leptospiruria and leptospires may be secreted in the urine for more than a month. Antibodies appear during the second phase, resulting in immunologic injury which may be responsible for the meningitis and uveitis.

Several severe outbreaks involving multiple people have occurred in the last 20 years. In the late 1970's, 11 milers on three Florida dairy farms became infected with *Leptospira hardjo* or *Leptospira pomona.* Employees from all three herds worked in waste-keep pits and were exposed to infected urine from the cows.

In a 1995 Nicaraguan outbreak there were 13 known human deaths and more than 2,000 sick. In addition to the generally recognized symptoms, hemorrhage and/or hemorrhagic pneumonitis was observed. The pulmonary involvement has not been reported previously in the Western Hemisphere, but had been observed in Korea and China. The source of the Nicaraguan infections were due to exposure to water and soil that had been contaminated with animal urine following heavy rainfall and flooding in the area. In 1996, 9 of 26 people became clinically ill after white water rafting in Costa Rica. Ingestion of, or submersion in, contaminated river water was suspected as the source of the leptospires. All of those infected recovered whether treatment with antibiotics was used or not. More recently in 1998, 74 of 639 triathalon participants had an acute febrile illness after prolonged swimming in a lake in Illinois, USA. Clinical signs and preliminary serologic testing indicates that this condition was leptospirosis. The leptospiral serovars implicated in these outbreaks were not reported.

### *Leptospirosis in Animals*

Leptospirosis is a systemic and/or reproductive disease in animals, and the outcome of the infection can vary with age and species.

*Canine*: In dogs, four clinical syndromes are generally recognized: acute hemorrhagic, icteric, subacute/uremic, and inapparent/subclinical.

Animals with the acute hemorrhagic syndrome (usually caused by *L. icterohemorrhagiae*) exhibit high fever, vomiting, prostration and generally die. Those with the icteric form (usually caused by *L. icterohemorrhagiae* or *L. canicola*) have icterus, depression, fever, and bloody feces and urine. The subacute or uremic form (usually caused by *L. canicola*) is characterized by extensive renal damage, ulcerative stomatitis, and death in a large number of cases. The inapparent or subclinical form (usually caused by *L. canicola* or *L. grippotyphosa*) normally only results in leptospiruria.

*Bovine*: Clinical conditions can range from leptospiruria, infertility, or decreased milk production (usually *L. hardjo*), to abortion in adults and neonate mortality (usually *L. pomona* and

*L. hardjo*), hemoglobinuria, icterus, and fever in calves (usually *L. pomona, L. grippotyphosa, and L. icterohemorrhagiae*).

*Porcine*: Infections are usually subclinical or asymptomatic, often with leptospiruria. Infertility, abortions, and stillbirth have been attributed to infections caused by *L. pomona, L. icterohemorrhagiae,* or *L. canicola.* However, infertility and delayed conception may be due to *L. bratislava* infections. High mortality may be seen in young pigs infected with *L. icterohemorrhagiae.* Other signs observed are metritis, icterus, anemia, fever, and meningoencephalitis.

*Equine*: Abortions due to serotype *L. pomona (L. kennewickii)* have been documented in several recent outbreaks in the United States. Clincal signs such as fever, anorexia and depression are occasioinally seen. Recurrent iridocyclitis, also known as "periodic ophthalmia", or "moon blindness", have been reported as sequelae to equine leptospirosis.

*Ovine*: Subclinical infections with leptospiruria (usually *L. hardjo*) have been reported. Sometimes acute disease caused by *L. pomona* and manifested by depression, dyspnea, hemoglobinuria, anemia, and high mortality occurs in lambs.

### *Diagnosis*

*Serology*: Because humans and animals produce predominately IgM agglutinins which persist for months after the onset of infection, serologic testing is the most practical means to diagnose leptospirosis.

Tests available are the microscopic agglutination test (MAT), ELISA, indirect hemagglutination, indirect fluorescent antibody, complement fixation, and the macroscopic plate agglutination test.

The MAT, using live leptospires, is the primary serologic test in use. The test is sensitive, serovar specific, and is primarily directed toward IgM but will detect IgG. The principal disadvantage of the MAT is the associated health risks for laboratory technicians. The other tests are not readily available for use with animals and are not routinely used in veterinary diagnostic laboratories. A commercial ELISA which detects IgM antibody in humans and is considered a suitable screening test for "early detection" is currently available from Australia and is in widespread use in humans. This ELISA has not been evaluated for use in animals.

The interpretation of serologic tests is difficult if the vaccination history of the animal is not known. Vaccination may result in an IgM antibody titer that persists for two to three months. Becaue vaccines contain multiple serovars, in some species positive MAT titers with three or more serovars in a single sample indicates likely use of vaccinations. In dogs, however, antibody titers to two serovars, i.e., *L. icterohemorrhagiae* and *L. canicola* may indicate recent vaccination.

Paired samples (acute and convalescent) are always preferred by diagnostic laboratories, but in many instances they are difficult or impractical to obtain from livestock. The most practical sampling method is to collect samples from at least 10 animals, or 10% of the animals in a herd. These should include samples from both affected and non-affected animals. This approach is usually preferred by the livestock producer if only from the standpoint of animal handling. In instances where only one sample is available, a titer equal to or greater than 1:800 to a single serovar with minimal to negative titers for other serovars would indicate the possibility of infection and should dictate further testing and/or antibiotic therapy.

An example of the use of serologic testing for diagnosis is manifested with reproductive problems in swine herds. The herds were unvaccinated, but several serum samples tested had titers to *L. bratislava* in the 1:100–1:800 range. The use of leptospiral bacterins that contain *L. bratislava* has been successful in correcting these reproductive problems.

Care shold be exercised in evaluating leptospiral titers in equine cases associated with abortion or uveitis. Many horse serum samples will react with high titers to multiple serovars, which makes interpretation difficult. Diagnosis of equine leptospirosis should be based on high serologic titers (greater than 1:6,400) or extensive microscopic examination (FA, histopathology, or dark field microscopy) of the fetus. A positive MAT titer or fetal fluid is significant.

Cattle infected with *L. hardjo* may remain subclinical, with delayed breeding and reproductive failure the only signs observed. In addition, antibody titers may be no higher than 1:100–1:400. In numerous herds, serologic testing of multiple animals has resulted in "low" titers only to *L. hardjo*. In these situations, in the absence of other etiologic agents, great economic losses due to leptospirosis can be occurring without any overt clinical signs being observed.

The incidence of chronic nephritis in dogs due to infection with *L. grippotyphosa* has increased. Since this serovar is not included in any of the canine bacterins, MAT titers of 1:200–1:800 to *L. grippotyphosa* in dogs are significant and should not be ignored.

*Culture*: Diagnosis of leptospirosis can be made also by culturing the organism from blood, urine, and tissue suspensions. Culture requires specialized media or animal inoculation, and contamination specimens require filtration or treatment with 5 fluorouracil. These techniques are time consuming and difficult for the inexperienced individual.

Blood for culture should be drawn during the febrile stage, i.e. between the second and eighth day of illness, and inoculated immediately into a suitable medium. This inoculated medium should be examined at weekly intervals for at least six weeks before called negative. A zone of growth in semisolid medium may be observed visually, but all cultures should be examined by darkfield microscopy.

Urine samples should be collected aseptically during the second week of illness, examined microscopically, and inoculated into culture media. If the urine cannot be cultured immediately, make a 1:10 dilution with 1% bovine serum albumin and transport at room temperature to the laboratory.

Tissues (kidney, liver, and brain) should be collected and refrigerated as soon as possible after death, then macerated and inoculated into culture media.

Laboratory animals such as hamsters, gerbils, and guinea pigs may be inoculated with specimens from infected animals when leptospiral numbers are low or severe contamination is a problem. Blood, urine, and tissue from these laboratory animals should be collected for culture.

*Direct examination*: Other methods for detection of leptospires in tissues or fluids include dark-field microscopy, silver staining, and FA examination. Care should be exercised in interpreting results when any of these microscopic methods are used alone.

### *Vaccination: Bacterins*

Commercial bacterins are approved for general use in cattle, swine, and dogs. Five serovars, *L. pomona, L. hardjo, L. grippotyphosa, L. icterohemorrhagiae,* and *L. canicola* are normally included in the cattle bacterin. An additional serovar, *L. bratislava,* is added to swine. The canine bacterin contains only *L. icterohemorrhagiae* and *L. canicola.* When properly administered, these bacterins can assist in prevention and suppression of clinical disease or outbreaks. Management of animals to control exposure to potential sources of leptospires, e.g., contaminated water or excessive rodent populations, is of utmost importance and will enhance the efficacy of bacterins. It should be pointed out that in many areas of the world, the serovars implicated in outbreaks or individual cases are not usually included in commonly used bacterins.

Bacterins initially produce primarily an IgM antibody response, which is indicated by a low MAT titer that may persist up to three months. However, the decline or lack of a MAT titer following vaccination does not indicate that the animal is not protected. Further procedures such as the hamster protection or growth inhibition tests using serum from the vaccinated animal can be done to validate protection. Revaccination produces only an IgM response which may result in higher and more persistent titers. Vaccination will not eliminate the carrier state, so once the control program is instituted on a farm it should be continued. All replacement animals brought onto the premises should be vaccinated according to the manufacturer's recommendation prior to contact with other animals.

*L. hardjo* infections in cattle can be especially difficult to control once the infection is established on the premise. In addition to the initial vaccination, boosters may need to be given at least every six months rather than the recommended annual vaccination.

### *Treatment*

In the acute stage of the disease, whether animal or human, therapy with Doxycycline, Penicillin, or Amoxicillin should be instituted immediately. Intravenous Penicillin or Ampicillin, with concomitant supportive therapy, should be used in critically ill patients. The prophylactic use of Doxycycline (200 mg weekly) is recommended in high-risk individuals, e.g., military personnel undergoing jungle warfare training. In addition, Tetracycline, Cephalosporins, Lincomycin, or Erythromycin have been used successfully for treatment.

If streptomycin or dihydrostreptomycin is available, these can be used to eliminate leptospires from the kidneys of animals, thus reducing the carrier state. Tetracycline also has been recommended. The use of these antibiotics has been especially valuable in infected herd bulls, dogs, or other valuable animals.

Leptospirosis will probably never be eradicated but with careful management, diagnosis, treatment and use of bacterins it can be controlled.

CHAPTER 9

# Chlamydia (Psittacosis, Ornithosis) in Birds and Humans

*By Dr. T. H. Eleazer*

### *Geographical Incidence*

The disease has occurred in many parts of the world and its appearance in any area would not be surprising considering the world wide movement of pet and exotic birds.

## HISTORY, CAUSE, CHARACTERISTICS

*Chlamydia psittaci* infection is a naturally occurring, contagious, systemic disease of birds, animals, and humans. This disease can be economically devastating to the poultry producers, because of condemnations at slaughter, egg production losses, the expense of antibiotic treatment to reduce mortality, morbidity, and reduce shedding of the organisms to a level that will allow safe marketing. It can also cause illness in humans. The disease was first reported in the 1930's in psittacine birds (cockatiels, parrots, parakeets, etc.) and humans. The classification of chlamydias has been a constantly changing saga and may continue to be, but for now it appears that they are eubacteria and that they represent a hitherto unrecognized eubacteria group. They are very small bacteria and are found inside the cells of infected hosts. The highest incidence of this disease continues to be in psittacine birds and in humans that come in close contact with these birds. Feces (dry and fresh) and respiratory secretions are the primary avenues for transmission. This organism has only 2 recognized species at present, *Chlamydia psittaci* and *C. trachomatis,* but this is likely to change as more chlamydial isolations are made and more precise methods for identification are developed. *C. trachomatis* occurs naturally in mice and humans, and *C. psittaci* is found in birds, animals, and can infect humans.

Chlamydia are very susceptible to chemicals that attack the fat content of the organism or the integrity of the cell wall. Even in the presence of a lot of tissue debris, the organisms are inactivated by surface active compounds such as quaternary ammonium compounds (quits) and fat solvents. The infectivity of Chlamydia is destroyed within minutes by exposure to common disinfectants such as benzalkonium chloride (Rocal, Zephiran), alcoholic iodine solutions, 70% ethyl alcohol, 3% hydrogen peroxide, and silver nitrate, but they are resistant to cresylic acid compounds and lime. 20% suspensions of infectious tissue homogenates are inactivated in 5 minutes at 56C, 48 hours at 37C, 12 days at 22C, and 50 days at 4C.

### *The Disease in Birds*

The principal vectors of Chlamydiosis are undoubtedly birds that are either inapparently infected carriers or secondarily infected birds that serve to amplify the spread of Chlamydiosis during migratory movements or during feeding time. The role of arthropods in the transmission of chlamydia is uncertain, although homogenates of mites from turkey nests have been shown to contain chlamydia. Simulid flies were suspected of spreading Chlamydia among turkeys in a South Carolina epidemic. Transovarian transmission from hen through the egg to the chick apparently does not occur. Chlamydia have been isolated from around 100 species of birds, but mostly from psittacines (especially cockatiels and parakeets). Some of the most important species involved in Chlamydiosis are:

*Turkeys*: Infection usually occurs naturally via inhalation, and the incubation period varies according to the number of Chlamydial organisms inhaled and the virulence of the infecting strain. Experimentally the incubation period may be 5–10 days or longer. Signs of infection with virulent strains of Chlamydia are loss of weight, loss of appetite, and fever. Infected birds excrete yellowish-green gelatinous droppings that usually soil vent feathers, and in laying hens egg production declines rapidly (birds laying 60% may drop as low as 10–20%) and in some cases may cease or remain low until the birds completely recover. Birds infected with less virulent strains of the organism usually go off feed, have loose greenish droppings, and egg production is less severely affected. At the peak of infection with a virulent strain of chlamydia, 50 to 80% of the birds may show clinical signs of the disease. If infected with a less virulent strain only 5 to 20% may show signs. Mortality usually ranges from 10 to 30% with the more virulent strains, and 1 to 4% with the milder strains. Of course, the earlier in the outbreak that treatment is started the less the mortality will usually be. Lesions seen in turkeys usually include diffuse congestion of lungs, fibrinous exudate in the pleural cavity, thickening and inflammation of the pericardium, and enlargement of the heart with thick fibrinous (whitish) plaques over the epicardial surface. Severe heart and lung damage is the usual cause of death. The air sacs are thickened and covered by fibrinous exudate and the spleen is enlarged, dark, soft, and may be covered with greyish-white spots. The more virulent the infecting strain of Chlamydia, the more severe the lesions tend to be.

*Psittacines*: Most reported cases of Chlamydiosis occur in psittacine birds, hence the common names Psittacosis, Ornithosis, or Parrot Fever. Psittacines may show only mild or no clinical signs, yet shed the organisms in their feces and nasal and eye secretions. Lesions, if seen, are much the same as seen in turkeys but are usually much milder and there may be only a slight conjunctivitis and nasal discharge. In many cases varying degrees of splenic enlargement may be the only lesion seen. Psittacines are viewed by the Centers for Disease Control (CDC) as by far the major threat to humans as far as chlamydia infections are concerned.

*Chickens*: Chickens are relatively resistant to chlamydia infections. Most natural cases are inapparent and transient. Serological surveys indicate that the incidence of infection is low.

*Ducks*: Chlamydiosis is not an important disease in commercial ducks in the USA, but it is in Europe, both economically and as a public health hazard, Internal lesions are similar to those seen in turkeys, but there is also a pronounced serous to purulent discharge from the eyes and nostrils that encrusts the feathers of the head. Morbidity usually runs from 10 to 80% and mortality can run 0 to 30% depending on age and the presence of concurrent infection with salmonellae.

*Pigeons*: Chlamydiosis is thought to be endemic in pigeon population and to be perpetuated primarily through a parent to nestling transmission cycle. Signs of infection vary, but those that develop acute disease lose their appetite, become unthrifty, and have diarrhea. Some develop conjunctivitis, swollen eyelids, and rhinitis with respiratory distress accompanied by rattling sounds. As the disease progresses, affected birds become weak and emaciated. Recovered birds become carriers of the organism without further signs of disease. Some birds go through infection without signs of disease other than possibly a transient diarrhea, and become carriers. Internal lesions, if seen, are similar to those seen in turkeys.

*Humans*: This disease in humans often causes influenza-like symptoms and can lead to severe pneumonia and non-respiratory health problems. However, with prompt proper treatment, the disease is rarely fatal.

From 1988 to 1997, the Communicable Disease Center in Atlanta, GA USA (CDC) received 766 reports of Chlamydiosis in humans in the USA. This is thought to be underestimated because Chlamydia infections are difficult to diagnose and therefore many cases go undiagnosed. Of the human cases reported to CDC, 70% were traced to exposure to pet caged birds and of these 43% were in fanciers and owners of pet birds and 10% were in pet shop employees. Others at risk included pigeon fanciers and people whose occupations place them at risk. For instance, there have been cases in turkey slaughtering plants in which turkeys with Chlamydia-like infections were processed.

Infection can also result from transient exposure to infected birds or their droppings. Because of this aspect, people not involved in "high risk" situations previously mentioned may be infected occasionally.

The editor is aware of a situation where people in a small office building became sick with acute and chronic respiratory infections which were much later diagnosed as Chlamydiosis. Epidemiological studies revealed large numbers of pigeons roosting in an area where intake for air conditioners took place.

The disease should be considered when humans are sick with an influenza like condition that does not follow the usual pattern or lasts much longer than expected or the sick person's history reveals one or more of the previously mentioned exposure factors.

### *Immunity*

Immunity to chlamydia is generally poor and short lived; however, there is age-associated resistance to infection as birds grow older.

### *Diagnosis*

This disease may be suspected using signs and lesions seen, but the diagnosis needs to be confirmed or denied by a veterinary diagnostic facility. The tissues of choice for finding chlamydia in fresh dead infected birds are air sacs, spleen, pericardium, heart, liver, or kidney. From live birds, cloacal swabs, feces, heperinized blood, conjunctival scrapings (if inflammation or exudate are present), and peritoneal fluid (if respiratory signs exist). An effective method of screening birds for chlamydia is to collect cloacal swabs, place them in a transport media obtained from a disease facility, and get into the laboratory for isolation or demonstration of the organisms as soon as possible.

### *Treatment and Prevention*

Chlortetracycline (CTC) is the drug of choice in treating chlamydia infections. A level of 400 grams per ton of feed or high level treatment in the drinking water should be used in turkeys. They should be treated for 2 weeks and then given no medication for 2 days prior to slaughter for human consumption. This treatment greatly reduces the shedding of chlamydia and makes carcass handling much safer.

Treatment regimens for other species, including humans, using CTC can also be worked out. Early and proper treatment is usually very effective in controlling clinical signs and shedding of the organisms, except in pigeons. Treatment is effective in alleviating clinical signs but does not eliminate the carrier state in pigeons.

Treatment in humans involves 2–3 weeks of taking a common, relatively inexpensive antibiotic called doxycycline by mouth. Alternative treatments are available for pregnant women or other persons such as children less than 8 years old, who should not take Doxycycline; Erythromycin is the choice in such persons. However, doctors may have received information about newer drugs as well. With appropriate treatment, fewer than 1% of persons with the disease will die from it. Untreated however, it can have a mortality of up to 20%. (From Psittacosis Question and Answer Sheet by Centers for Disease Control and Prevention-Revised 6–95).

If Chlamydia infection is suspected, workers and/or handlers who must work with or around these birds should wear protective masks and clothing and use good personal hygiene such as thorough hand washing and disinfection.

### *References*

The information in this article was obtained from personal experience of the author and from Diseases of Poultry, published by the Iowa State University Press, Ames, Iowa 50010.

***Editor's Notes***

Other recent sources of material on Chlamydiosis are as follows:

*Compendium of Chlamydiosis* (Psittacosis) control 1999. As published in the Journal of The American Veterinary Medical Association, Vol 214, No. 5, March 1999. The material was developed by Psittacosis Compendium Committee, National Association of State Public Health Veterinarians.

*Detection of Chlamydiosis in a Shipment of Pet Birds, Leading to Recognition of an Outbreak of Clinically Mild Psittacosis in Humans* by John F. Moroney, etc. presented at the 36th Interscience Conference on Antimicrobial agents and Chemotherapy Sept. 1996 and Reprinted by CDC.

## CHAPTER 10

# Listeriosis in Animals and Humans

*By Dr. Raymond K. Hines*

### *Introduction*

Listeriosis is a disease that has three basic clinical forms. The clinical presentation may be encephalitis, abortion, or septicemia. *Listeria monocytogenes* is the bacteria that causes Listeriosis. The organism can infect at least 47 species of animals and 22 avian species, including rabbits, guinea pigs, gerbils, chickens, sheep, goats, cattle, foxes, swine, chinchillas, ferrets, raccoons, horses, *and man.* The disease produced by *Listeria monocytogenes* varies with the species of animal infected, however, monocyte leukosis is universal. In poultry, including chickens, turkeys, and ducks, the primary lesion is myocarditis and liver necrosis. In rabbits, chinchillas, guinea pigs, and gerbils, the primary lesion is focal necrosis of the liver. In ruminants, clinical representations are one of the three forms: abortion, encephalitis, or septicemia.

## HISTORY

An organism that caused a generalized infection with a monocyte leukocytosis in rabbits and guinea pigs was discovered by Murray, Webb, and Swann, while working in England in 1926. The organism had not been previously described, and was named *Bacterium monocytogenes.*

In 1927, Pirie, in South Africa, found a new bacterium to be the cause of "Tiger River Disease". This disease caused focal necrosis of the liver in gerbils. Pirie could not classify the bacteria to a suitable genus. He suggested that the name *Listerella hepatolytica* be used in honor of Lord Lister. Pirie knew his organism to be similar to the isolate of Murray, Webb, and Swann. Pirie suggested the name be *Listerella monocytogenes,* if they were identical. The 1934 Bergey's Manual listed the name as *Listerella monocytogenes.*

In 1948, the name was changed to *Listeria monocytogenes* to end confusion with the plant genus *Listerella.* The disease name automatically changed from listerellosis to listeriosis.

## *Listeria monocytogenes*

*Listeria monocytogenes* can be found growing in soil, vegetation, *streams,* sewage, and in a *carrier state* from clinically normal animals. If not ubiquitous, *Listeria monocytogenes* is at least extremely wide spread.

The organism is a small gram positive coccobacillus. *Listeria* has a tumbling motility on a wet mount when grown in liquid media at room temperature (20° C). If cultured at higher temperatures (37° C), the tumbling motility is greatly reduced. Motility is also seen as a characteristic "umbrella" pattern forms from a stab on motility media incubated at room temperature. The colonies are small, translucent, gray, and have a close halo of ß hemolysis on blood agar media. The organism tests positive for the CAMP test, is esculin positive, and catalase positive, but is $H_2S$ negative on TSI. Growth of the organism can take place at temperatures from 4 to 44° C (refrigeration temperature is 4° C).

## *Geographical Distribution*

Listeriosis occurs world wide. It can be found in developing countries and extremely rural areas, but also occurs in developed countries with elaborate sanitation schemes, including those in North America and Europe.

### *Listeriosis in Man*

#### A. Disease

Listeriosis can be characterized as producing variable clinical presentations depending on the species of animal affected. Some of the common symptoms are monocyte leukosis, fever, encephalitis, focal necrosis of organs especially hepatic necrosis, and abortion. Many species can be apparently normal carriers. Means of transmission include transplacental, at birth during passage through the birth canal, by drinking contaminated milk or contaminated water, by inhaling contaminated dust, and from infected animals and sewage.

#### B. Food Borne Threat

Listeriosis has become one of the hot topics of food borne "emerging" diseases. Contamination with *Listeria monocytogenes* has been one of the primary reasons for product recall within the United States. One of the big outbreaks occurred in California through soft Mexican-style cheese. In the making of the cheese, a milk starter culture is inoculated with the fermenting organism. After an incubation period, the starter culture is added to a larger vat of milk. In this case, the cheese was made from pasteurized milk, however, the cheese maker used unpasteurized milk for the cheese starter culture. Hard cheeses go through salting and aging processes, both of which reduce the growth of microbes. Hard cheeses have been found to be *Listeria* free. There have been reported cases of listeriosis caused by contaminated cabbage. The cabbage had been fertilized with animal feces. *Listeria* has been found in fresh rainbow trout and other fish. In the last few months, numerous meat products were found to be contaminated with *Listeria monocytogenes.* The U.S. Department of Agriculture's Food Safety Inspection Service has issued recalls for 85,000 pounds of bacon bits and bacon pieces distributed over fifteen states. Cooked luncheon meats, including wieners and summer sausage, were recalled in Ohio. Roasting sausage was recalled in New Jersey. Hot dogs were recalled in Pennsylvania.

Hams were recalled in Michigan. There has been a recall of luncheon meat from a nationally known company, and the death of a man has been associated with it.

The wide spread use of refrigeration, the convenience of semi-cooked foods, and the use of microwave cooking have increased the risk of getting listeriosis. The problem with microwave cooking is that the heat is not uniform. Foods heated in the microwave have hot and cold areas. Heat kills *Listeria*, but the entire portion must be heated thoroughly. Another factor is the increased practice of eating at restaurants, cafes, and fast food establishments. In commercial food preparation, several factors increase the risk of food borne infection. First, the amount of ingredients is greatly increased, increasing the possibility of introducing contamination. Secondly, food is often prepared ahead of time and reheated prior to being served, allowing the proper time and temperature for bacterial growth. Finally, training for food handlers in food safety is usually minimal, increasing the risk of contamination through human error. The most at risk are pregnant women and people with weak or compromised immune systems, such as the elderly, infants, chronically ill people, people infected with HIV, and people taking chemotherapy.

### C. Prevention

Because of risk to pregnant women, the Australian New Zealand Food Authority advises, through its pamphlet "Listeria and Pregnancy," that pregnant women avoid certain foods. The advice equally applies to other people at risk. They advise pregnant women to avoid soft cheese (Brie, Camembert, ricotta), ready cooked cold meats (roast or boiled), ready cooked chicken, pate, ready made salads (salad bars, packaged salads), and raw or smoked seafood (raw oysters, sashimi, sushi, and chilled or frozen smoked seafood). Several products should be added to this list, including hot dogs, frankfurters, or wieners that are not cooked well done and served while still hot. All cold meat products such as luncheon meat, bologna, or other cold sausages should be avoided. Raw unpasteurized milk from any species should never be consumed.

It is recommended that fresh fruits and vegetables be washed and dried before eating. *Listeria monocytogenes* can be killed by thoroughly cooking; however, the food should be eaten while hot. Water can be an important means of transmission of the disease. Impure water can be treated by boiling 10 minutes, or by filtering then adding 0.02 parts per million (ppm) of calcium hypochlorite. If the water has organic material or is cloudy, add 0.05 ppm calcium hypochlorite.

**D. Treatment**

Antibiotic susceptibility testing should be done on all isolates of *Listeria monocytogenes.* Traditionally the treatment has been to give high levels of ampicillin or penicillin given I.V. for 3 to 6 weeks.

### *Listeriosis in Cattle and Goats*

**A. Disease**

In cattle and goats, there are three forms of the disease: encephalomyelitis, abortion, and septicemia. Usually the disease has a low morbidity with small numbers of affected animals; however, herd outbreaks are known to occur. Most veterinarians are familiar with "circling disease" of cattle and goats, the encephalitic form of the disease. The clinical symptoms are a manifestation of the pathologic change of focal necrosis in the caudal brainstem and occasionally the cerebellum. Clinical signs include fever, anorexia, depression, and proprioceptive deficits. Dropped jaw, drooped ear, and facial anesthesia may be seen. Nystagmus may occur. Stertorous breathing and dysphagia are often present. As the disease progresses, circling or uncoordinated movement may occur. The other major presentation in cattle is septicemia and late term abortion. Respiratory infections caused by *Listeria monocytogenes* have been seen in feedlot cattle. *Listeria monocytogenes* can cause keratoconjunctivitis in cattle and sheep. The sheep's eyes are often also infected with *Branhamella ovis.*

Ruminants become infected through the eyes, nose, and mouth. The mechanical vectors may be from vegetation, infected dust, feces, or from infected silage. Herd outbreaks often result from eating infected silage. If the pH of the silage does not get below 4.6, *Listeria* can grow. Contamination of feed bunkers by goats playing in the bins has been seen.

### B. Prevention

The proper ensiling process prevents the growth of *Listeria.* Corn silage should be made from corn cut in the early dough stage, properly chopped, tightly packed in airtight storage, and fermented at least three weeks. If there is any doubt about quality of the silage, the pH should be tested, and the silage should be cultured for *Listeria.*

Aborting animals should be separated from the rest of the herd. The organism may be present in high numbers in feces, aborted fetuses, birth fluids, milk, and newborn animals.

### C. Treatment

Antibiotic susceptibility should be done if possible. Oxytetracycline and penicillin have been used to treat infected cattle. For treatment to be effective, it must be given early, in very high doses, and for a prolonged period of time.

## *Listeriosis in Poultry*

### A. Disease

In pigeons, listeriosis causes septicemia or encephalitis. Septicemia occurs most often. Older pigeons are noticeably depressed, and die rapidly. Younger pigeons have a higher incidence of disease, but the disease does not progress as fast. Young pigeons are depressed, become emaciated, and have the fading bird syndrome. The encephalitic form of disease is characterized by birds walking in circles, muscle tremors, and toricollis.

At necropsy, common symptoms are myocarditis, focal necrosis and enlargement of the liver and spleen. Signalment seen to a lesser degree are peritonitis, enteritis, and salpingitis. Other findings include evidence of emaciation. Chickens and other poultry are affected in the same way.

**B. Control**

Control of the disease in poultry involves finding the source of the infection and getting rid of it. Any build-up of old or moldy vegetation, feed, and litter should be removed. After cleaning houses and pens, disinfection should be done. One method of disinfecting soil or wood is to treat it with an acid solution. Solutions with a pH of 3.5 or less will kill *Listeria.*

Because poultry can be long term carriers of *Listeria monocytogenes,* housing for them should be separate from other farm animals.

**C. Treatment**

Antibiotic susceptibility testing should be done. The tetracyclines have been used to treat infected birds, however, antibiotic resistant strains of *Listeria monocytogenes,* have been found in birds.

### *Listeriosis in Other Species*

In swine, listeriosis is not an economically important disease. Pigs do occasionally develop the disease. Affected pigs are stiff legged in the front, but may be uncoordinated or drag the rear legs.

Encephalitis in foxes resembles rabies or distemper infections. Listeriosis must be a rule out for encephalitic foxes.

Listeriosis is rare in horses; however, encephalitis and septicemia have been reported.

### *Listeriosis in Humans*

In man, the disease almost always involves the central nervous system. Symptoms may also include shock, a red rash over the lower portion of the body and circulatory collapse. Infants and elderly are particularly susceptible to the infection. The disease is potentially fatal.

Treatment is with antibiotics, such as penicillin. It must be started early and continued until several days after the symptoms disappear.

### *Recent Advances in Diagnosis of Listeria*

*Listeria* is sometimes very difficult to culture. Feces, cerebrospinal fluid, blood, amniotic fluid, placenta, and genital tract specimens should be cultured. Trypticase soy sheep blood agar and Columbia base Colistin Nalidixic Acid (CNA) agar are used for culture. The organism will grow under aerobic conditions, but grows better under microaerophilic conditions.

When culture on ordinary media is negative, cold enrichment should be done. Cold enrichment is done making a one to ten dilution of the test material in trypticase soy broth or tryptose broth, refrigerate (4° C) for up to two months, and subculture weekly on solid media.

The difficulty of culturing *Listeria monocytogenes* has resulted in specialized pre-enrichment media to enhance growth. Some of the specialized media are Fraser Broth; *Listeria* Enrichment Broth; *Listeria* Enrichment Broth, FDA; *Listeria* Enrichment Broth I, USDA FSIS; *Listeria* Enrichment Broth II, USDA FSIS; *Listeria* Fermentation Broth; Mcbride Agar, Modified; and McBride *Listeria* Agar.

With increased interest in culturing food products for *Listeria,* new media combinations and formulations are being developed. Food samples tend to have low numbers of contaminating organisms. Because of the low numbers of organism per gram of product, larger sampling sizes are necessary.

One protocol uses 25 grams of food sample. The sample is added to 225 mL of Buffered Peptone Water, stomached, and incubated overnight. One mL of the Buffered Peptone Water is then added to Fraser broth with Ferric ammonium citrate additive. After another overnight incubation, the media is streaked onto Modified Oxford Media and Blood Agar Plates. Modified

Oxford Media has esculin which is hydrolyzed by *Listeria*, turning the media dark brown to black. On Blood Agar Plates, *Listeria* has small white colonies with a halo of ß hemolysis.

The USDA protocol uses 25 grams of food sample added to 225 mL of University of Vermont *Listeria* Enrichment, stomached, and incubated overnight at 30° C. One ml of the broth is then added to Fraser broth with Ferric Ammonium Citrate and incubated overnight at 37° C. The next step is to streak the sample onto Modified Oxford Media and on Horse Blood Overlay Agar, and incubate at 37° C for 24–48 hours. Positive organisms are inoculated into brain Heart Infusion broth and incubated at 35° C for 24–48 hours.

Positive organisms from either of the above protocols are *Listeria*, but must have ancillary tests to confirm that the species is *L. monocytogenes*. *Listeria monocytogenes* is catalase positive, ß-hemolytic, CAMP test positive, L-Rhamnose positive, Mannitol negative, and D-Xylose negative. *Listeria monocytogenes* ferments glucose, trehalose, and salicin.

### *Summary*

Listeriosis is a disease found in many different animals and bird species, with symptoms that vary with the animal. The clinical disease types are encephalitis, abortion, and septicemia. Listeriosis is caused by *Listeria monocytogenes*, a small gram positive coccobacillus that does not form spores. The organism is highly mobile when grown at room temperature, is catalase positive, hydrolyses esculin. *Listeria monocytogenes* will grow at a wide range of temperatures, including refrigeration temperature, but high heat or low pH (acid) will kill it. Pregnant women, the elderly, infants, and people with compromised immune systems are at risk and should avoid certain foods.

CHAPTER 11

# Roundworms in Animals and Humans

*By Dr. Prema Arasu*

## *Roundworm Parasites in Animals and Preventing Human Infection*


### *Summary*

*Toxocara* ascarids and hookworms are the 2 most common intestinal parasitic nematode (roundworm) infections of dogs and cats. Both of these parasites also have zoonotic health implications and can cause visceral and cutaneous larva migrans in humans. This article will address the biology and life cycle of these parasites as well as the control and treatment of infection in animals and in humans. While there are related ascarid infections in other domestic animals (e.g. *Parascaris equorum* in horses, *Ascaris suum* in pigs, *Toxocara vitulorum* in cattle, *Ascaridia* sp. in chicken/turkeys), these are not typically associated with zoonotic disease. Similarly, the relatively common human parasite, *Ascaris lumbricoides*, is not infective to animals. However, *Baylisascaris* sp. that normally infects wildlife can cause severe visceral larva migrans in a wide range of other hosts including humans, and will be briefly discussed.


## HISTORY AND GEOGRAPHICAL INCIDENCE

*Toxocara* species roundworms and *Ancylostoma* species hookworms are common nematode (Greek for 'Thread or Round Worm') parasites of the small intestine of dogs and cats. They have a worldwide distribution particularly in temperate, tropical and sub-tropical regions. In some parts of the world, infection rates approaching 100% have been reported in some populations of puppies.

There are 2 major species of interest with *Toxocara* roundworms: *T. canis* in the dog (and other canids), and *T. cati* in the cat (and other felids). There is also a related parasite, *Toxascaris leonina,* which can infect both dogs and cats but it is not zoonotic and will not be discussed here. In contrast to these ascarid worms, there are several different hookworm species and the prevalence of each species varies with the geographical area. The species of interest are: *Ancylostoma caninum* in canids (rarely in felids), *A. braziliense* in canids and felids, *A. ceylanicum* in canids and felids, *Uncinaria stenocephala* in canids and felids, and *A. tubaeforme* in felids.

### *Biology*

*Toxocara* sp., sometimes loosely referred to as the "the common roundworm," are thick, white robust looking worms belonging to the ascarid group of nematode parasites. Adult parasites reside in the small intestine and reach a length of 1–2 inches. Mature female worms are prolific egg producers and generate as many as 200,000 eggs a day that are eliminated into the environment in the animal's feces. With intestinal burdens of few to several hundred worms, infected animals can easily contaminate the environment daily with millions of eggs. Ascarid eggs are round and have a thick, brown outer coat that is sticky and also protects the embryo from harsh environmental conditions. Within the protective egg coat, the *Toxocara* embryo requires 2–4 weeks to divide and develop into the infective larval stage. Because of the protective outer coat, "infective eggs" can persist for months to years. This "infective egg" must be ingested by a host for further development to occur. The time from infection to detection of

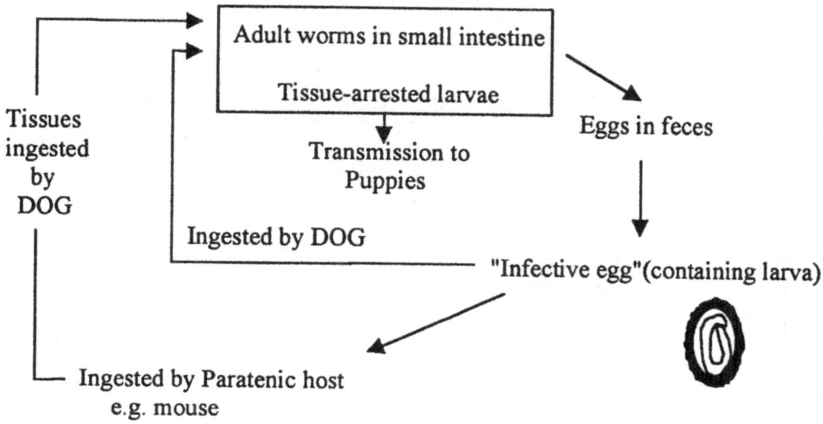


***FIGURE 1.*** **Life Cycle of *Toxocara canis*, DOG host.**

eggs in the feces is called the pre-patent period and ranges from 3–5 weeks. The representative life cycle is shown in Figure 1.

*Ancylostoma* sp. hookworms are also found in the small intestine and can reach an inch in length. These hookworms have a large mouth that is bent or "hooked" and contains 2 or 3 pairs of sharp teeth that are used to anchor onto the intestinal wall and pierce underlying blood vessels (Note: *Uncinaria* sp. have cutting plates instead of teeth). As with *Toxocara*, adult worms mate in the small intestine and eggs produced by the female worm are released in the feces of the host animal. A single *A. caninum* adult female can produce as many as 16,000 eggs per day. Under warm, moist, well-aerated conditions, cell division occurs and the infective larvae hatch from the eggs in 5–7 days. These larvae can persist in the environment for weeks to months under mild conditions but are rapidly killed by direct sunlight or freezing temperatures. The free-living larvae must be ingested or penetrate the skin of a suitable host for further development to occur. From the time of infection, the pre-patent period for detection of eggs is about 2–3 weeks. The representative life cycle is shown in Figure 2.

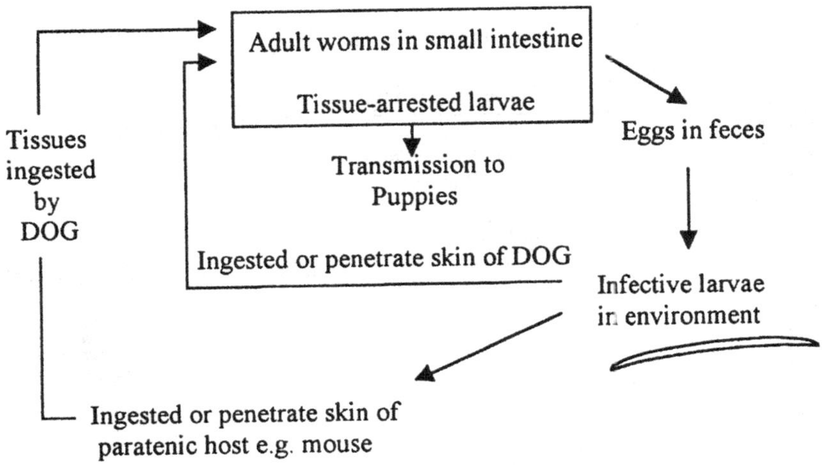


*FIGURE 2.* **Life cycle of *Ancylostoma caninum*, DOG host.**

## *Transmission Routes*

The varied and highly efficient transmission routes are the major cause for the high prevalence of the intestinal roundworms. Five major routes are described.

1. By ingestion of "infective eggs" or larvae in the environment

"Infective eggs," or larvae, are ingested by dogs or cats, which are the usual definitive hosts for these parasites. In the small intestine of the animal, the larvae (which have to hatch from the egg in the case of *Toxocara*) penetrate the wall of the intestine, migrate to the lungs, enter the trachea and are coughed up, swallowed and returned to the small intestine. Here, they complete development to become sexually mature adult worms. In a very young puppy or kitten, most of the larvae will become adult worms in the small intestine.

However, for yet unknown reasons, in a mature dog or cat, many of the larvae reaching the lungs will enter the blood circulation and be distributed throughout the body to different organs and distant tissue as "arrested" larvae until they receive signals to reactivation during pregnancy or stressful situations.

2. By skin penetration (hookworms only)

Hookworm larvae that penetrate the skin migrate extensively and may cause dermal lesions. Larvae that finally reach the small intestine will mature to adulthood and those that do not will encyst in the tissues as arrested larvae pending reactivation.

3. By ingestion of the larval-infected tissues of a "paratenic" host

Animals other than dogs or cats may also ingest the *Toxocara* eggs or hookworm larvae, or hookworm larvae in the environment may penetrate their skin. In these so-called paratenic hosts (e.g. mouse, rabbit, earthworm, etc.) the larvae are unable to develop normally and remain encysted as arrested larvae in the tissues. If these tissues are eaten by a dog or cat, the larvae are released, reactivated and continue normal development to become adult worms in the small intestine.

4. By transplacental migration into the fetuses. (*T. canis* in dogs)

During pregnancy, specific signals are apparently received by the tissue-arrested larvae, which are stimulated to reactivate. The reactivated larvae can either migrate to the small intestine of the mother or into her developing fetuses. Therefore both the newborns and the mother (lower probability) will have active intestinal infections.

5. By transmammary transfer to the nursing offspring

Pregnancy induced reactivation of arrested larvae also results in migration of the parasites from various locations in the body to the mammary tissue (or to the small intestine of the mother). Larvae in the mammary gland then transfer with the milk into the intestine of her nursing offspring and mature into adult worms. This is well documented with *A. caninum* hookworms as well as with *T. cati* in the cat; with *T. canis* in the dog, transmammary transmission does occur but to a much lower extent than transplacental transmission of the larvae to the fetal pups.

### *Pathology and Clinical Disease*

Within the dog or cat, the migratory stages of the *Toxocara* or hookworm larvae cause some level of inflammation in the tissues traversed, especially the lungs. With heavy infections, young animals may display respiratory signs. However, adult worms in the small intestine are the major cause of clinical disease.

With the large *Toxocara* worms, heavy infection interferes with normal digestion and absorption of nutrients. In addition to obstruction of the lumen of the intestine, the host mounts immunological and inflammatory reactions to these foreign agents. The animal therefore shows signs of enteritis (inflammation of the intestine), diarrhea and subnormal growth. Infected dogs and cats may appear malnourished, undersized, and lethargic, have poor hair coats and be prone to other disease. Loss of protein due to intestinal damage contributes to fluid accumulation in the abdomen (ascites) and a "pot-bellied" appearance. The pathology caused by *Toxocara* infections in dogs and cats is quite similar to the pathology and clinical signs of *Ascaris lumbricoides* infections in children.

With the blood-feeding hookworms, host animals primarily suffer from iron deficiency anemia. As they feed, hookworms secrete an anticoagulant to prevent the blood from clotting which results in freely bleeding areas when they change to a different attachment site. (A note of interest: the gene from this parasite-specific anticoagulant has been cloned and is being used in studies on human blood clotting disorders). A newborn puppy with 50–100 adult *A. caninum* worms may easily lose enough blood to reach life-threatening condition because young animals do not have a competent bone marrow system to quickly replenish lost cells. Heavily infected animals have pale mucous membranes, and liquid feces that are dark in color from partially digested blood.

Another clinical sign associated with the skin-penetrating *Ancylostoma* and *Uncinaria* hookworm larvae is dermatitis. Lesions are usually noted in the inter-digital spaces and may extend up the limbs, but generally subside in less than a week.

### *Immunity*

Because of the transplacental and transmammary routes as well as environmental routes of infection, almost all dogs and cats have an early history of infection with these parasites. As a result, most animals probably develop some level of acquired immunity to subsequent episodes of infection. It is rare to find an adult animal with signs of disease or a high fecal egg count unless the animal is compromised by other infections, is malnourished or has a weak immune system.

### *Diagnosis*

Since parasite eggs are shed in the feces, diagnosis of an active infection is usually rewarded by a positive fecal flotation test. *Toxocara* sp. eggs are round, have a thick, rough coat and contain single ova as is typical of the ascarid family (Figure 3). Hookworm eggs are oval and contain a morula of cells i.e. the embryo has begun cell division and reached the 2, 4 or 8 cell stage (Figure 4). This appearance of the hookworm egg is also described as "strongyle-type" because it is similar to those of other related parasites (e.g. the common parasites of horses, cattle and sheep). In some instances, dogs that eat the manure of these later-mentioned animals can display high numbers of "strongyle-type" eggs which pass through in their own feces and may be mis-diagnosed for an active hookworm infection! Additionally, fresh

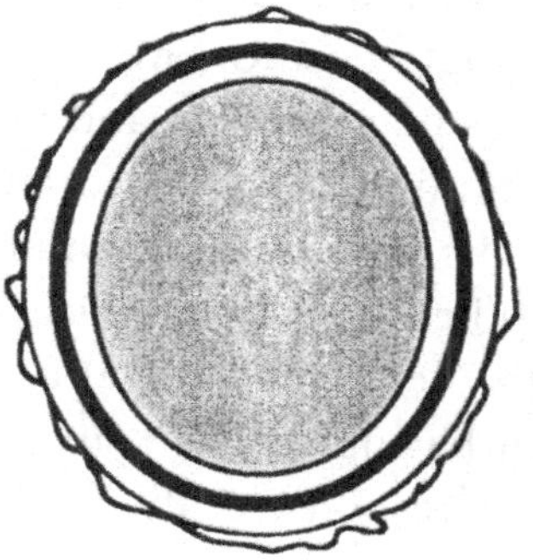

***FIGURE 3.*** ***Toxocara* sp. egg (~ 75–90 microns long).**

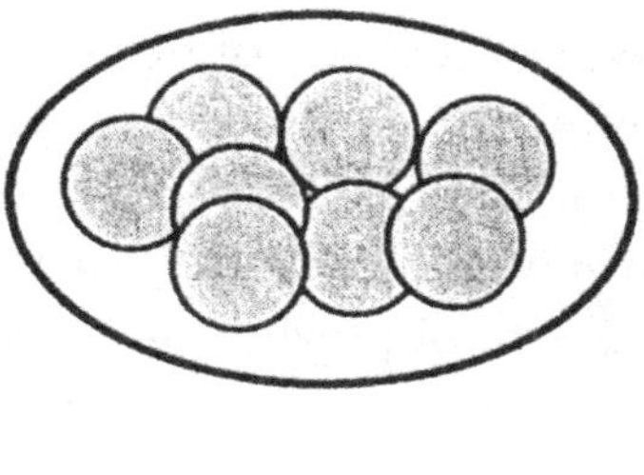

***FIGURE 4.*** **Hookworm egg (~ 55–80 microns long).**

feces should always be used in diagnostic tests; this is because hookworm eggs can rapidly develop and hatch to release the free-living infective larvae giving a low or negative fecal egg count. Hookworm larvae cannot be easily distinguished from other types of non-parasitic larvae normally present in soil.

In some instances, both *Toxocara* and hookworm infections may not be diagnosed in the face of active infection and disease if the parasites have not reached sexual maturity and are not producing eggs. This is a common finding with young animals that have acquired the infection from their mothers and display severe signs of parasitic infection but have negative fecal test results.

### *Treatment*

There are many effective drugs available as tablets, granules and liquids for elimination of intestinal stages of *Toxocara* and hookworms in dogs and cats. These include drugs such as the Benzimidazoles (e.g. Fenbendazole), the avermectins (e.g. Ivermectin, Milbemycin Oxime), Pyrantel, and older generation drugs such as Dichlorvos, Disophenol and N-Butyl Chloride. The drugs may be administered as a single dose or over a range of days, or in a periodic or continuous manner. Age and weight of the animal as well as ease of administration determine the choice of drug. Repeated treatments are crucial in animals that are heavily infected. It should also be noted that clinical disease may not be supported by a positive fecal test; immature worms may be causing pathology without having reached sexual maturity and in these cases, a strategy of "response to therapy" should be implemented.

While many drugs are available for treatment of intestinal stage infections, the tissue-arrested larval stages of both *Toxocara* and *Ancylostoma* are somewhat refractory to the effects of most drugs. Very high doses of some of the avermectins (e.g. Ivermectin or Doramectin) are effective in reducing the transmission of larvae from the dam to her fetuses or pups when administered during pregnancy, but this is still not a routine practice. As a result, the general recommendation is to treat puppies and kittens, as well as their dams, soon after delivery.

Newborn puppies and kittens are particularly susceptible to the pathogenic consequences of intestinal parasites and should be treated immediately upon suspicion of disease. Supportive therapy such as fluids and a good diet are also beneficial. These young animals at 1–3 weeks of age will have negative fecal tests because the pre-patent periods of the parasites have not been reached. In the case of hookworm disease, some puppies may even require blood transfusions and iron supplementation. Drugs used in very young animals should be carefully monitored for adverse side effects and toxicity. Pyrantel and Fenbendazole are generally used in these situations. Veterinarians may administer anthelmintics to pups as early as 2 weeks of age and to kittens as early as 3 weeks of age to ensure the good health of the growing animal as well as prevent environmental contamination. Treatment usually continues on a bi-monthly schedule until the animal reaches 2–3 months of age.

With the current practice of using heartworm preventative in some parts of the world with *Dirofilaria immitis* infections (mosquito transmitted parasite that causes heart and lung disease), many dogs and cats receive supplemental drug doses that also eliminate the intestinal roundworms e.g. Pyrantel plus Ivermectin or Milbemycin formulations.

### *Human Disease*

The increase in dog and cat ownership in many countries, the high prevalence of infection in both pets and stray animals, the widespread environmental contamination and, in particular, the play habits of children all combine to result in frequent opportunities for zoonotic transmission of these parasitic infections.

How do people get infected? The sticky, hardy infective eggs of *Toxocara* may be accidentally ingested, e.g. by children playing in dirt, by improper washing of fruits and vegetables that have been in contact with contaminated soil, and various other unhygienic practices. With hookworm larvae, infection more typically occurs by skin penetration e.g. walking barefoot or lying on sandy beaches or public places that are contaminated. Not surprisingly, plumbers, electricians and gardeners who work on their hands and knees are more susceptible to these larval infections.

What are the signs of infections? In humans, the parasites *rarely* reach the intestine and develop to adult worms; rather, the larvae migrate abortively in the tissues and the symptoms of pathology and disease (called "larva migrans") depend on which particular tissue or organ is reached. In most cases, the infective dose is low, and the infection is asymptomatic and goes undetected.

With *Toxocara* larvae hatch from the ingested eggs and migrate extensively throughout the body resulting in **Visceral Larva Migrans** especially in liver, lungs, kidneys and brain. "Ocular larva migrans" is the term used when the eye is infected by these migrating larvae causing a granulomatous retinitis. Larvae migrans can be caused by a number of nematode parasites. Clinical signs depend on the site of pathology and may include severe inflammation, fever, enlarged liver, asthma or pneumonitis, loss of or impaired vision, and in a very few cases, death. A serological test for antibody response to the parasite is available in the U.S.; about 1,000 cases are identified a year. The choice of treatment depends on the signs and tissues infected. Drugs typically used for treatment belong to the benzimidazole group e.g. thibendazole or mebendazole. With ocular lesions, treatment is dependent on the exact location of the parasite as drugs could exacerbate the immuno-pathological response to the dying worm.

With hookworm larvae, penetration of unprotected skin causes **Cutaneous Larva Migrans** or "creeping eruption." Similar lesions may be induced by fly larval stages or other parasites such as *Strongyloides* sp. (Many different species and hosts; *S. stercoaralis* can transmit from dogs to cause a chronic infection in humans), *Bunostomum plhebotomum* (hookworm of cattle), *Gnathostoma* sp.

(parasite of carnivores), as well as the species of hookworms that normally infect man (*A. duodenale, A. ceylonicum, Necator americanus*). In a previously sensitized individual, the larvae migrate in the dermis producing red, wavy tracks that are very itchy, and typically, the parasite is 1 to2 centimeters ahead of the inflammatory lesion. If not treated with topical or oral benzimidazoles, the larvae usually die within weeks to months. In some instances and particularly with heavy infection, hookworm larvae may penetrate and cause lesions in deeper tissues and organs.

*A. caninum* induced **gastroenteritis** has been clearly documented in Queensland, Australia, and other cases have been reported in various regions including the Philippines, South America, Israel and the U.S.; the sharp abdominal pain of sudden onset is caused by the occasional larva which reaches the small intestine and matures to adulthood. A patent infection (i.e. production of parasite eggs) is not typical and cannot be used as a diagnostic technique in humans. Response to treatment with mebendazole is usually immediate.

### *Prevention and Control*

Pets should be routinely examined for parasites and treated with appropriate anthelmintics. Since the eggs of these intestinal worms are not infective until a suitable incubation period has elapsed, feces should not be allowed to accumulate in the environment or public areas, and certainly, one should avoid walking barefoot or lying in areas that may have been previously contaminated with the feces of infected animals.

Can infected areas be decontaminated? The ascarid eggs of *Toxocara* are sticky and highly resistant to many chemicals so that it is hard to kill eggs in soil. A 1% sodium hypochlorite (bleach) solution is usually effective in stripping the outer egg coat so that they can be washed off the floors and walls. The eggs also deteriorate if exposed to full sunlight or desiccation. Hookworm larvae are much more susceptible to dryness and are easily inactivated by bleach. With concrete or cement-covered areas, high powered water jets or hot water applications are also effective. Fecal material should be removed on a regular basis and appropriately discarded.

### *Zoonotic Implications of Baylisascaris sp. Infections*

*Baylisascaris* sp. (e.g. *B. procyonis* in raccoons, *B. columnaris* in skunks, etc.) is an ascarid parasite (similar to *Toxocara* sp.) that typically infects wildlife hosts. However, domestic animals and humans that have contact with wildlife and accidentally ingest the "infective eggs" of this ascarid, can develop a serious form of visceral larva migrans. In aberrant hosts, *Baylisascaris* larvae tend to migrate and invade the central nervous system. Because they also grow in size as they migrate, the pathology and resulting clinical disease is generally serious and can be fatal. Hay, straw, or other feeds that are contaminated with the eggs of this parasite are a typical source of infection; additionally, attics or feed storage areas that may be frequented by wildlife should be avoided as play areas by children.

CHAPTER 12

# Tapeworms and Trichinosis of Farm Animals which Can Cause Problems in Humans

*By Dr. Keith Flanagan*

## CYSTICERCOSIS: HISTORY AND REVIEW OF THE LIFE CYCLE

Cysticercosis is caused by the ingestion of eggs of the *Taenia* tapeworm. This is more common in developing countries because sanitation facilities are lacking and animals are allowed to roam freely, having access to human feces. It is also seen more frequently in areas where beef and pork are eaten raw or insufficiently cooked. Prevalence is highest in parts of Latin America, Africa, Southeast Asia and Eastern Europe.

The definitive host (host that harbors the adult parasite) for both bovine cysticercosis (*Taenia saginata*) and swine cysticercosis (*Taenia solium*) is man. The adult tapeworm in humans occurs after the ingestion of the encysted larvae from insufficiently cooked beef or pork. The infection of an adult tapeworm is called *taeniasis*. People infected with an adult tapeworm may expel several segments of the tapeworm daily. Each segment contains over a thousand eggs, which can survive for a month in water and up to six months in the grass or soil. These eggs are immediately infective and can then be ingested by cattle or swine, resulting in clinical cysticercosis. *Taenia solium* is considered a much greater public health threat than *T. saginata.* This is because *T. solium* eggs, when ingested by humans, can develop and encyst in the brain, often causing serious health problems (*Neurocysticercosis*).

Cysticercosis is generally more common in rural areas. However, a tapeworm carrier in a highly overcrowded urban area may represent an even more dangerous source of cases than in a rural area, especially if that person works as a food handler.

### *Clinical Disease in Animals*

Cysticercosis in beef cattle (beef measles) and swine (pork measles) rarely causes any clinical signs and usually goes undetected until slaughter. Severe infections may cause muscle swelling and pain, especially in the neck and tongue. Paralysis of the tongue may occur. On rare occasions, the larvae of *T. solium* may encyst in the brain of a pig, causing seizures or other neurological signs. Cysticercosis causes a great economic loss due to condemnation or reduced value of meat at slaughter.

### *Clinical Disease in Humans*

Adult tapeworm infections in humans may often go undiagnosed with few clinical signs. These signs may include abdominal discomfort, nervousness, loss of appetite, insomnia, weight loss and diarrhea. Sections of the tape worm (proglottides) may be observed in the feces. These appear as short, flat, white segments that, when dry, look much like a grain of rice.

Cysticercosis, or infection by the larval form, is a totally different disease and can be fatal. The larval form tends to encyst in the brain tissue. Cysts can cause a wide variety of symptoms, depending on where they locate in the brain. In many developing countries, cysticercosis is the major cause of seizures. Other symptoms may include headaches, blindness, incoordination, and loss of motor function. The cyst may also locate in the heart, lung, muscle or just under the skin. Muscle pain and intense itching may be observed with the latter two forms.

### *Animal Diagnosis*

Serological testing can also be done in animals, but is usually too expensive to be feasible. Cysticercosis is usually discovered during slaughter. However, about 80% of the infected pigs will have visible cysts on the ventral surface of the tongue. These cysts will appear as 0.5–1 cm, shiny, fluid filled nodules. This visual examination may be useful for field screening and survey work. In the carcass, cysts are most often found in the muscles of the jaw, neck, tongue, diaphragm, heart, shoulder, and thigh.

### *Human Diagnosis*

Adult tapeworm infection can be diagnosed by identification of the segments or the eggs in the feces under a microscope. Obtaining the scolex (head) of the tapeworm following treatment confirms the diagnosis and assures the elimination of the worm. Usually, only one worm is present. Specific serologic tests should support the clinical diagnosis of cysticercosis. These tests are expensive and usually not available in developing countries. Subcutaneous cysts may be visible or can be palpated as 0.5–1 cm nodules just under the skin. Microscopic examination of an excised cyst confirms the diagnosis. Internal cysticercosis can be diagnosed by an MRI or CAT scan.

### *Control and Eradication*

Due to life-threatening and debilitating consequences of human neurocysticercosis, control measures should be implemented in endemic areas. In theory, the life cycle of cysticercosis should be easy to break, and the disease easily controlled. However, due to lack of education about the disease, poor sanitation practices, and long standing animal husbandry practices, control and eradication may be a long time in coming.

As with any disease, education of the population is essential prior to any other control measures being implemented. The population must be aware of the dangers of the disease as well as the life cycle of cysticercosis. Personal hygiene must be stressed in both the public schools as well as in adult education classes.

Improved personal hygiene would decrease the risk of human-to-human transmission of eggs. Increased access to improved sanitation facilities is essential in preventing animals from having access to human feces. There is a direct correlation between the incidence of cysticercosis and the lack of latrine facilities. Raw sewage should not be used for fertilizing or irrigating fields. Composting human waste for six months to a year kills the eggs and renders it safe as fertilizer.

Improved animal husbandry practices are essential. If animals are not allowed access to human feces, the life cycle can be effectively broken. Even with education, these changes will be slow in coming. Pens are expensive to build and free ranging animals are easier and cheaper to take care of.

The parasitic disease discussed in this paper, as well as many others affecting both animals and man, cause untold suffering and economic loss in much of the world. Though poorly understood in the past, animal disease and parasite problems with human implications have long been with us. They have been extensively studied in this century and are now well understood. Many of these problems can be greatly lessened and even eliminated. There are several basic steps that are well within the reach of most individuals. In other cases, community efforts are necessary. Successful control and prevention programs have been carried out in many areas of the world.

1. ***SANITATION***
   - Prevent humans from coming into contact with the feces of other humans.
   - Prevent animals, especially dogs and pigs, from contact with human feces.
   - Measures that prevent human exposure usually take care of this problem. Preventative plans are available in most countries, from international agencies such as the United Nations and many other organizations. In temporary situations, such as campsites where building materials are costly or not available, trenches or small holes can be dug and covered. They must be

deep enough to prevent animal access and some distance from the drinking water source.

2. ***COOK ALL MEAT FOR HUMAN CONSUMPTION UNTIL WELL DONE***
   - In order to kill organisms in meat it must be cooked to 55° C and until at least gray in color with no reddish areas remaining or thoroughly boiled for at least thirty minutes. This will help in the prevention of other diseases such as Tuberculosis.
3. ***DON'T FEED UNCOOKED MEAT SCRAPS TO ANIMALS***
   - Any source of meat scraps, from slaughter houses, restaurants, hospitals and airports as well as household waste should be thoroughly cooked to kill the causative organisms of parasitic and disease problems. Bones protect the organisms and are a problem which requires a prolonged procedure. This is especially true of not feeding any meat to dogs which has not been fully cooked. As well, any raw meat of any kind should not be left where wild animals may have access to it.
4. ***QUICK BURIAL OR BURNING OF DEAD ANIMALS***
   - This is necessary to ensure that other animals do not have contact with the carcasses and spread the disease.
5. ***INSPECT MEAT PRODUCTS AT SLAUGHTER PLANTS***
   - Though not possible in many areas, this is one of the most important measures.

### *Summary*

**THE MORE OF THESE PRACTICES THAT CAN BE CARRIED OUT THE GREATER THE CHANCE OF IMPROVING HEALTH AND LIVING CONDITIONS.**

Proper handling of infected meat is also a critical step. Inspection and condemnation of infected meat is effective in decreasing the incident of disease, but often the infrastructure is not in place to carry this out. Freezing infected meat at –10° C for four days will kill the cyst. This is rarely possible in developing countries. Cooking the meat at temperatures of 45–50° C will also effectively kill the cysts. Salting or pickling of the infected meat is not effective in killing the cysts.

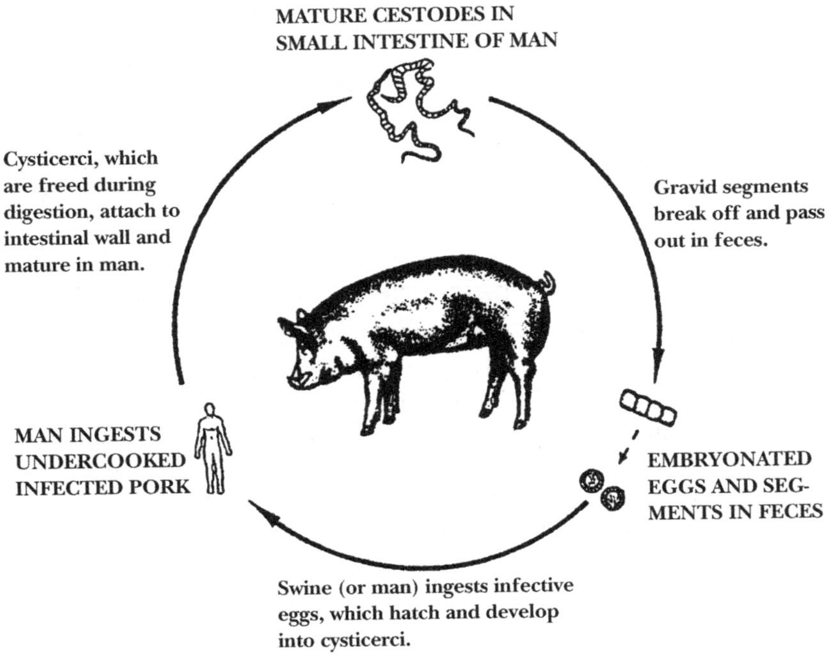


**Life Cycle of *Taenia Solium*, the Pork Tapeworm.**

Mass treatment of the human population in an area endemic for cysticercosis would also be beneficial toward control and eradication. This would be expensive and would only be effective if other control measures were implemented at the same time. Several isolated cases of human neurocysticercosis have been recently identified in developed countries. Most of these cases have occurred because of poor sanitary hygiene practices of *Taenia* positive food handlers. Most of these food handlers have been immigrants from *Taenia* endemic areas. An adult worm may remain in the intestine and continue shedding eggs for up to 30 years. The eggs can remain viable in the environment for months. Testing and treatment of selected individuals, especially those preparing food, should be considered for controlling human cysticercosis.

### *Animal Treatment*

Until recently, treatment of animals for cysticercosis has not been economically feasible. Praziquantel given to pigs at a dose of 50 mg/kg daily for 15 days was effective, but could cost up to U.S. $200.00. Albendazole given at 30 mg/kg daily for 3 days was also effective. The cost is almost U.S. $20.00 per treatment. A recent study using a single dose of oxfenazole at 30 mg/kg showed great promise at a cost of about U.S. $1.20. Further studies need to be documented to confirm these findings.

### *Human Treatment*

Both Praziquantel and Albendazole are being used for the treatment of both taeniasis and cysticercosis in humans. If either disease is suspected, one should contact his or her physician for proper diagnosis and treatment.

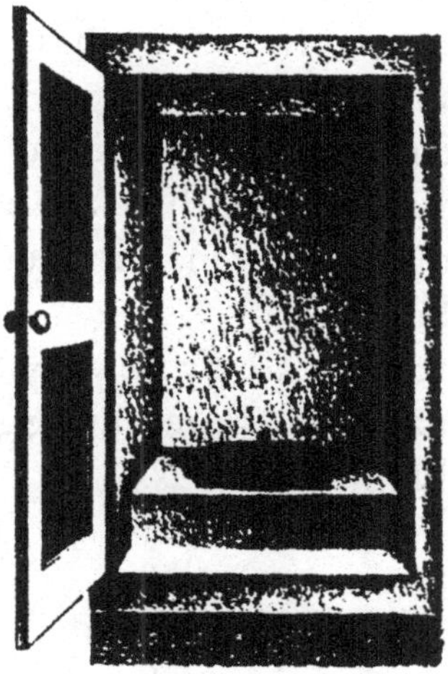

Drawing of an outside sanitary facility-latrine. There are many variations of this design and many other designs which are satisfactory. All of them incorporate the following:

- Enclosed to keep out flies and other insects.
- A roof to keep out rainfall that might cause the pit to overflow.
- A cover over seat to keep flies and insects from access to feces in the pit.
- A pit under the facility for feces.

### *Other Tapeworms of Farm Animals That Can Cause Problems in Humans*

There are a number of tapeworm species in farm animals that can cause problems in humans. In sheep and goats, and at times in cattle, several species of Moniezia can cause problems in humans. They are found world wide where cattle, sheep and goats are raised.

In the life cycle of these tapeworms, animals grazing on infested pastures pick up the eggs which hatch in the intestines. They then migrate through different organs and sometimes muscles on the way back to the intestines where they mature. Some of the migrating embroys encyst in the brain, spinal cord, internal organs and muscle.

Humans become infested by eating meat, especially brain and spinal cords and internal organs which are not fully cooked. The eggs hatch in the intestines and mature there. The mature tapeworms pass eggs in the feces.

Control and prevention are by fully cooking any *meat* of the animals eaten by humans and by preventing grazing animals from coming in contact with human feces.

### *Echinococcus*

Echinococcus granulosis is another tapeworm found in farm animals that can cause serious problems in humans as well as farm animals. The disease is called Hydatid Disease or Hydatidosis.

It is found worldwide where dogs run with farm animals. It is an infestation of the liver, lungs and occasionally the peritoneal cavity wall. It is caused by the larval stage of the tapeworm Echinococcus.

Dogs are the principal hosts of the adult worms. They do little obvious harm to the dog in most cases.

*Life Cycle* (see drawing of the life cycle at the end of this article). Sheep cattle, rodents, deer and humans, especially children, can become infested with larvae by ingesting eggs shed in the feces of infected dogs.

Humans can also become infested by eating raw meat containing the cysts.

After ingestion by the animals and humans, the eggs hatch in the intestines and the larvae travel through major blood vessels to the liver and lungs. The embryos then begin to form cysts in the organs and occasionally the peritoneal cavity wall as well. The larvae cause damage as they enlarge over a period of years.

### *Symptoms in Animals*

Symptoms in ruminants are non-specific and resemble those seen in many other conditions. They include unthriftiness, poor hair coat, vague digestive disturbances including constipation, mild diarrhea and dysentery. They are much more noticeable in animals less than six months of age, and they may also show noticeable stunting and become "pot bellied."

### *Symptoms in Humans*

Lung cysts cause coughing and chest pain. Liver involvement causes pain and eventually jaundice due to blockage of bile ducts. Infection of cysts leads to abscesses in up to 20% of cases. Bone cysts, less often seen, cause fractures and damage to bone tissue, and heart involvement leads to irregularities of heart beat and inflammation of the heart covering (pericarditis). Allergic reactions may occur from leakage of cyst fluid. Itching, fever and rashes are frequent.

### *Diagnosis in Ruminant Animals*

This is done at slaughter and by post-mortem examination. The cysts may be very obvious to the naked eye. However not all can be seen as some are very small and some are not on the surface of the organs.

### *Diagnosis in Humans*

This is done by x-rays, computed (CT scans), and ultrasound. Blood tests are available, but up to 50% of patients have negative results. Examination of aspirated cyst fluid for the parasites has been done, but carries the danger of a fatal allergic reaction. Skin tests are also used for diagnosis.

### *Treatment in Ruminants*

This is seldom done because of the cost and the difficulty of diagnosis in the live animal.

### *Treatment in Humans*

Treatment depends on the size and location of cysts as well as the symptoms they are producing. Surgical removal of cysts and surrounding tissue is the accepted method of treatment. However it carries a risk of cyst rupture with spread of allergic reactions. Some recent studies using medication along with aspiration and drainage of cysts instead of surgery, are encouraging. At present, medication alone only results in a low percent recovery rate.

## *Methods of Control and Prevention*

1. *Any method that prevents dog feces from contaminating* human food or drinking water. Any type of latrine for human waste would be very helpful in preventing the problem.
2. *Fully cooking all meat products used for food by humans.* In many cases the obvious cysts are removed from affected organs and the remaining meat is not fully cooked. This is detrimental because not all cysts are visible to the naked eye.
3. *Fully cooking meat product being fed to dogs.* The worst possible thing that is done is to feed the removed cysts to dogs. This is often done.
4. *Do not allow wild animals to have access to raw meat products.*

5. *Do not allow dogs and wild animals to have access to carcasses of dead animals* which often have the cysts in organs. As with any diseased carcasses, they should be disposed of promptly by burial or burning to prevent access of animals to the carcass.
6. *Development of more slaughter houses with veterinary inspection* to detect affected carcasses. Waste food products from slaughter houses are especially dangerous because they often include condemned parts.
7. *Ideally, though not practical, is the periodic treatment of dogs in an area.* This, with the elimination of stray dogs and extra dogs with the family that are not needed for herding animals and security, can be a big help. Periodic treatment of dogs in an area has been successful in a number of areas.

### *Summary*

**All of the above are very important, although not all are practical in many areas. Fully cooking all meat products used for human consumption and prevention of contamination of humans' food and drinking water by dog feces are probably the most important and practical methods. We must fully cook all meat products fed to dogs. As much education of families as possible about the information in this article and the article on the pork tapeworm should be done, especially aspects of prevention of infestation of animals and humans to help emphasize that we must fully cook all meat used for human consumption. In addition, other diseases of animals such as tuberculosis are also prevented to a great degree by fully cooking all meat products.**

*You may notice* that we have repeated some of the information on prevention and control of these parasites; that was done to emphasize the importance of these measures as well as to keep the flow of thought in case one should read only parts of the article.

*Notes on the drawing of the Life Cycle of Echinococcus*

1. You will notice that ruminants and humans can become infested when their food and drinking water are contaminated with dog feces.

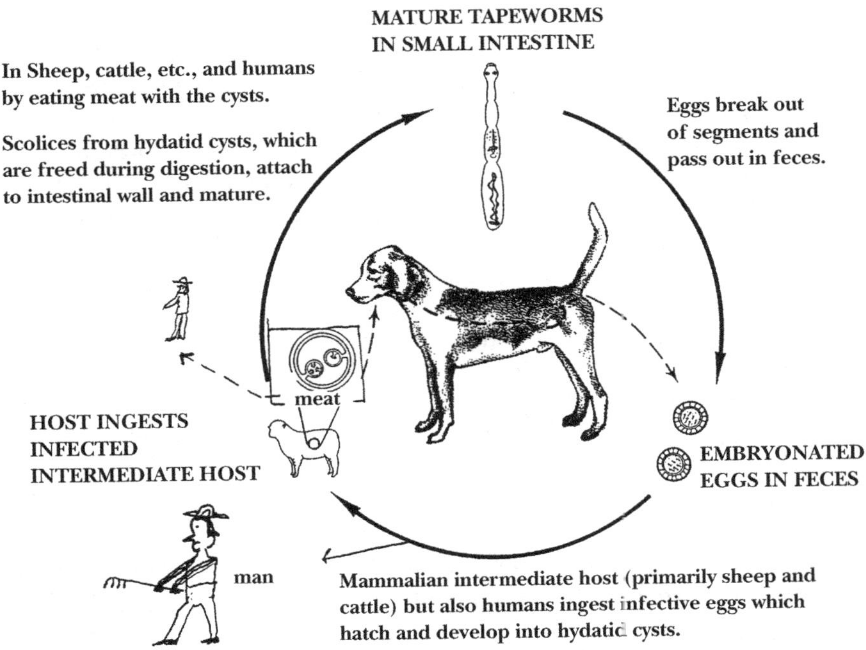


*Echinococcus granulosis Life Cycle.*

2. You will also notice that dogs and humans can become infested when they eat meat not fully cooked that contains the cysts. In most cases it is wise to assume that all ruminant meat is infested with the cysts.

## *Trichinellosis (Trichinosis)*

Trichinosis is a disease caused by the intestinal round worm (nematode) *Trichenella spiralis* whose larvae migrate to and become encapsulated in the muscle. It is normally a disease of swine, dogs, cats, rats, and many wild animals, including fox, wolf, bear, polar bear, wild boar and marine mammals in the Arctic. The hyena, jackal, lion, and leopard may be infected in the tropics. It is transmitted by eating raw or insufficiently cooked flesh of animals containing viable encysted larvae. Contaminated pork products are the most common source of infection for man. The larvae develop into adults in the epithelium of the small intestine. The mature female worms then produce larvae, which travel throughout the body and form cysts in the muscle tissue.

Clinical signs often appear 8–15 days after ingestion of infected meat and start with the sudden appearance of muscle soreness and pain. Edema of the upper eyelids and soreness are common and characteristic signs. Hemorrhage and pain of the eyes often follows. Thirst, sweating, chills and weakness follow the ocular signs. Remittent fever up to 40°C is common. Cardiac and neurological complications may appear during the third to sixth week. Death due to heart failure may occur either very early on, or between the fourth and eighth week. Serological tests and an increase in eosinophils may be helpful with the diagnosis.

Human trichinellosis occurs world wide, but its incidence varies depending on the practices of eating and preparing insufficiently cooked pork or wild animal meat. Thoroughly cooking the meat so that all parts reach at least 77° C or until the meat changes from pink to gray will insure safety. Freezing meat at –15° C for 20 days will also effectively kill the cyst.

The feeding of raw or improperly cooked garbage to swine especially around towns and cities is a major source of trichinosis. The garbage from hospitals and airports and seaports is especially dangerous.

Where garbage feeding (outside one's own household source) has been outlawed or the cooking of the garbage tightly inspected, trichinosis has become a minor problem. However, in other areas it continues to be an area of concern. This is especially true of the feeding of raw slaughter house waste to swine.

In most situations where swine are raised, the cooking of all raw meat scraps and garbage greatly lessens this problem. *It also helps reduce human problems from Tuberculosis and many other conditions that are spread from raw meat.*

If trichinosis is suspected, one should consult his or her physician for proper diagnosis and treatment. Allergic reactions to the dying larvae may cause complications during treatment.

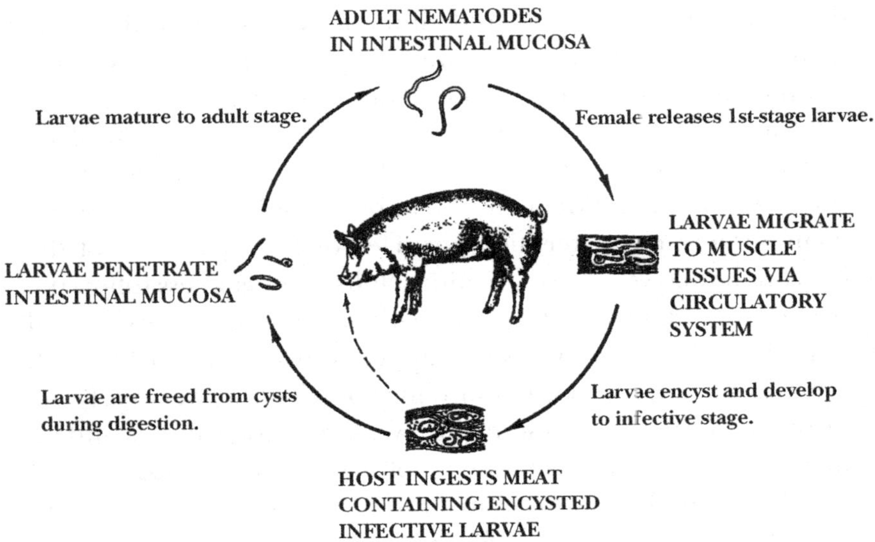


**Life Cycle of the *Trichinella spiralis*, the causative agent of Trichinosis in man.**

### *Human Infection With the Fish Tapeworm*

Information on the tapeworm of fish is included for your information. It reinforces the importance of fully cooking any meat from any source.

### *Diphyllobothriosis (Broad or Fish Tapeworm Infection)*

This is a human intestinal infection caused by the adult tapeworm, *Diphyllobothrium latum* or *D. pacificum*. Symptoms are usually trivial or absent. In long standing cases, vitamin B12 deficiency anemia may develop. Massive infections may be associated with diarrhea and obstruction of the bile duct or intestine.

This disease is most common in subarctic, temperate and tropical zones where eating of raw or partly cooked fresh water fish is common. Through this practice, humans are infected by the infective larval stage of the tapeworm. It then develops into an adult within the intestine and attaches to the jejunum, where it matures and starts laying eggs. The eggs are contained in segments of the tapeworm and are passed in the feces where they can contaminate fresh bodies of water. These eggs hatch and infect copepoda (tiny crustaceans) which are the first intermediate hosts. The infected copepoda are then eaten by freshwater fish. It is the infective stage in the fish that is infective for humans. It takes 3 to 6 weeks after ingestion of the infected larvae until there is a passage of the eggs in the stool.

Education about the disease and its life cycle is important. Cooking fish at 56° C for five minutes or freezing for 24 hours at –18° C insures protection. Dogs, bears, and other fish-eating mammals are also reservoirs. Consequently, breaking the life cycle in nature would be almost impossible.

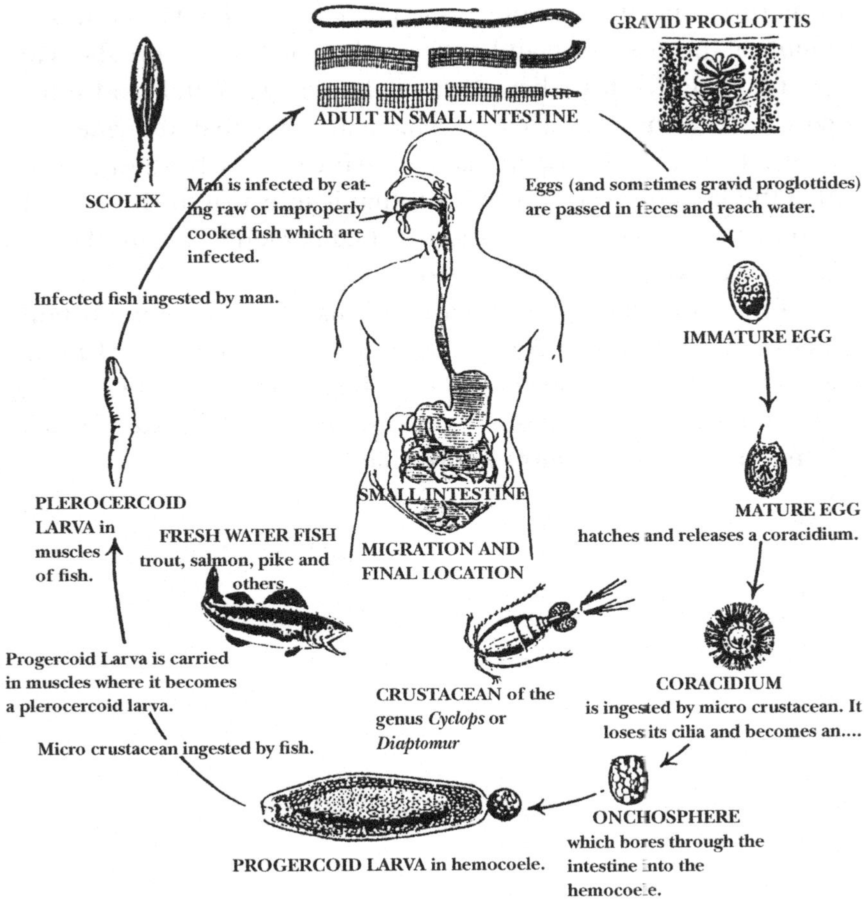


**Life Cycle, *Diphyllobothrium latum,* The Fish Tapeworm.**

# About The Authors

**Dr. Prema Arasu**
Dr. Arasu is a veterinarian and has a Ph.D degree in Parasitology. She works in the Department of Parasitology and Microbiology at North Carolina State University, USA, College of Veterinary Medicine in Raleigh, North Carolina.

**Dr. John R. Cole**
Dr. Cole is a medical microbiologist who is retired from the University of Georgia, USA Veterinary Diagnostic Laboratory at Tifton, Georgia.

**Dr. Russell W. Currier**
Dr. Currier is Environmental Epidemiologist and Public Health Veterinarian with the Iowa, USA Department of Health.

**Dr. Thomas H. Eleazer**
Dr. Eleazer is retired from Clemson University, South Carolina, USA as a poultry pathologist and Field Veterinarian. He is now a poultry disease consultant.

**Dr. Mitchell Esse**
Dr. Esse serves with The Veterinary Services of the United States Department of Agriculture as a regional specialist for Tuberculosis. He works out of Denver, Colorado, USA.

**Dr. Keith Flanagan**
Dr. Flanagan is a native of Oklahoma, USA. He is a veterinarian who practiced rural community veterinary medicine in that state. He is a long time field worker for Christian Veterinary Missions in Haiti and has done consulting work with missionary groups in other countries.

**Dr. Raymond K. Hines**
Dr. Hines is a veterinary microbiologist at the Clemson, South Carolina, USA Animal Diagnostic Laboratory in Columbia. He was formerly in mixed veterinary practice and retired from the Veterinary Corps of the U.S. Army.

**Dr. John C. Morrill, CVM, Ph.D.**
Dr. Morrill is Commander of the South Plains Veterinary Command of the U.S. Army at Fort Hood, Texas, USA. He served as World Health Organization consultant in the investigation of the Rift Valley Fever outbreak in Egypt in 1993.

**Dr. David S. Peterson**
Dr. Peterson has a Ph.D degree in Parasitology. He is an assistant professor in the Department of Microbiology and Parasitology in The College of Veterinary Medicine at The University of Georgia, USA.

**Dr. Venaye P. Reese**
Dr. Reese is a veterinarian with the Clemson University Livestock-Poultry Health Division in South Carolina, USA. She serves as Equine Programs Coordinator and has been involved in Equine veterinary practice.

**Dr. David Warner**
Dr. Warner works with The Veterinary Services of the United States Department of Agriculture. He has worked as the Brucellosis Epidemiologist for the Southeast Region of the U.S. and provided consultation in program development in Puerto Rico, Egypt, Mexico, Peru, Chile and Bolivia.

## Christian Veterinary Mission (Publisher of this book)

**Our vision is to see**

*Christ's love expressed through veterinary medicine.*

**Our mission is to**

challenge, empower and facilitate veterinarians to serve through their profession, living out their Christian faith.

CVM also provides education and encouragement for those who desire to minister through service, prayer, relationship building, and modeling Christ's love.

**About CVM**

Christian Veterinary Mission (CVM) is a registered non-profit Christian Service Organization 501(c)(3) based in Seattle, Washington, U.S.A.

CVM was founded in 1976 by Dr. Leroy Dorminy who came to realize the impact that veterinarians could have by integrating their faith with their practice, both locally and around the world. In 2008, CVM had nearly 30 veterinary professionals serving full-time internationally and over 200 veterinary professionals and student volunteers serve on short-term cross-cultural mission trips annually. CVM sponsors fellowship & prayer breakfasts at over 20 U.S. veterinary meetings each year and reaches out to veterinary students through Christian Veterinary Fellowship (CVF) groups in every veterinary school in the U.S. by encouraging them in spiritual growth and professional development.

There are over 3,500 veterinarians affiliated with CVM in the U.S. CVM also partners with organizations and networks in other countries that are focused on empowering Christian veterinarians. CVM has a volunteer advisory board of veterinarians who guide its vision, mission, and programming.

CVM books and the free International Animal Health Newsletter were written with small farmers, veterinarians, and agricultural development workers in mind. Our desire is that they would help individuals and groups develop an appropriate livestock program to meet community needs. CVM's Endowment Fund was started in the early years of the organization's life. The fund provides for meaningful programs that could not be funded by the regular budgeting process.

Made in the USA
Monee, IL
19 October 2026

66036207R00075